Writing a Medical Research Manuscript

Nicholas G. Zaorsky

Writing a Medical Research Manuscript

Springer

Nicholas G. Zaorsky
Department of Radiation Oncology
Mayo Clinic Florida
Jacksonville, FL, USA

ISBN 978-3-032-20275-8 ISBN 978-3-032-20276-5 (eBook)
https://doi.org/10.1007/978-3-032-20276-5

This Springer imprint is published by the registered company Springer Nature Switzerland AG
The registered company address is: Gewerbestrasse 11, 6330 Cham, Switzerland

Foreword

The advancement of medicine depends not only upon discovery but also upon dissemination. Scientific insights that remain confined to laboratory notebooks, institutional databases, or conference hallways do little to improve patient outcomes. It is through the disciplined craft of writing that research achieves its highest purpose by informing practice, influencing policy, and enhancing the health of individuals and communities worldwide.

For many trainees, junior faculty, and even seasoned investigators, the process of writing a medical research manuscript can appear opaque and daunting. From identifying a meaningful project and cultivating a productive mentoring relationship to structuring the introduction, methods, results, and discussion with clarity and rigor, each step requires intention and skill. *Writing a Medical Research Manuscript* offers a practical roadmap that guides readers through this complex but rewarding journey.

Zaorsky has meticulously organized a critical resource that reflects the true lifecycle of scholarly work. It begins with foundational elements of academic productivity, such as finding a mentor, defining a project, engaging coauthors, and crafting a prospectus. It then examines the essential components of the manuscript itself, providing clear guidance on reviewing the literature, presenting results effectively, constructing tables and figures, and composing precise abstracts and titles. The author also addresses the responsible use of modern tools, including reference managers and artificial intelligence, to enhance clarity and efficiency while maintaining scientific integrity. The final section demystifies the submission and publication process by outlining journal selection, common errors, peer review dynamics, response letters, and strategies for publicizing one's work.

Importantly, this text extends beyond technical instruction. It emphasizes professional values that are central to academic medicine, including integrity in authorship, clarity in communication, respect for reviewers, and stewardship of the scientific record. Practical checklists and structured guidance fill a gap that is often insufficiently addressed in formal training programs.

This resource will benefit a broad spectrum of learners, including medical and/or graduate students undertaking their index scholarly project, postgraduate trainees seeking to translate clinical observations into publishable research, and early-career faculty building academic portfolios. Experienced investigators will also find value in refining and actually strengthening their approach to writing and publication. This book is indispensable for medical and scientific institutional libraries—full stop. Moreover, academic departments and training programs would be wise to make this book readily accessible to their learners and faculty.

In an era marked by accelerating discovery and expanding technological tools, the need for thoughtful, methodical, and ethical scientific writing has never been greater. Zaorsky has created a concise and accessible guide that transforms an intimidating process into a manageable and empowering endeavor. By equipping investigators to communicate their findings effectively, this book advances medical science and, most importantly, improves patient care.

Charles R. Thomas Jr., MD
Geisel School of Medicine
Hanover, NH, USA

Preface

The purpose of this book is to teach medical researchers how to write a research manuscript, with the intent of it being published in a peer-reviewed journal. The book is organized into three parts.

(1) "The project and involved parties" discusses what the researcher should consider before starting a project.
(2) "The manuscript" discusses how each section of the research paper is written.
(3) "The submission and publication" discusses how to submit the manuscript to a research journal, make revisions, and publish the work.

There are short checklists of what to do at each part of the process. The book is meant to be brief and to help people get publications efficiently.

Q: Why do we, as clinical researchers, publish manuscripts?
A: There are two problems with medicine: (1) In 100 years, half of it will be proven to be false. (2) We don't know which half.
Manuscripts are the method that allows professionals to present their research findings to other professionals, with the goal of broadening scientific knowledge and discerning fact from fiction. If a researcher makes a discovery but is unable to communicate it effectively, the discovery does not advance society's scientific knowledge.
Another reason has become more apparent since the 1980s: promotion and tenure, which often influence salary.

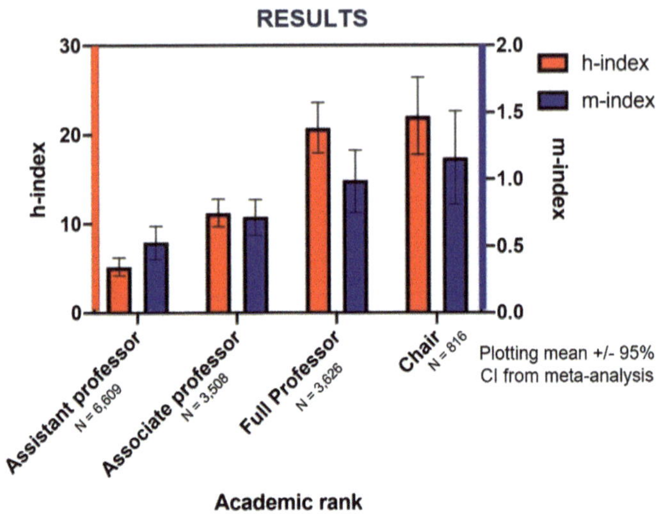

Figure. Publication metrics per academic rank (adapted from Zaorsky, 2020)

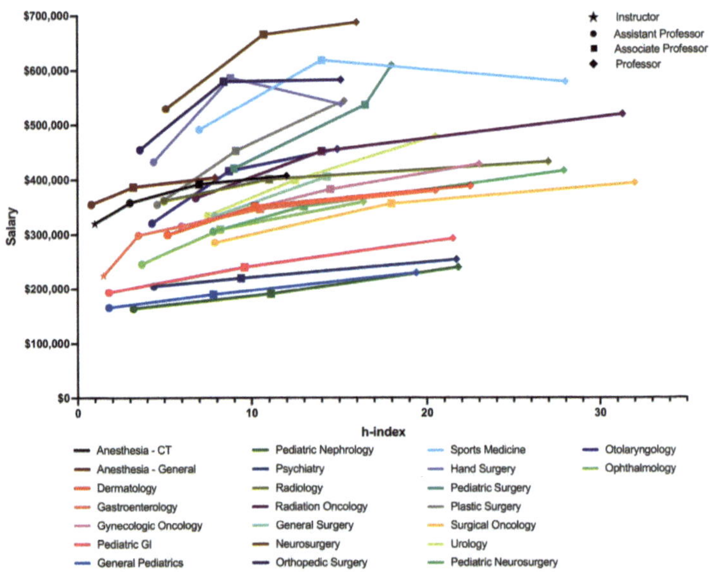

Figure. Average salary (in 2018, per AAMC and MGMA) per rise in h-index, with average h-index per academic rank (adapted from Zaorsky et al, unpublished work)

Q: What is the history of this book?

A: For background, when I worked with students on writing manuscripts as a resident in radiation oncology (2013–2017) and then junior attending (2017–2020), I used to give them a talk on how to write papers. Since I was giving it so often, I made it a slide set and instruction guide. In 2021, I figured I might as well help all trainees around the world, so I started posting on social media via Twitter. The talks were related to specific parts of writing a manuscript. This book summarizes the posts and presents them from start to finish, with an additional ~40% of unpublicized content.

Q: Do you need to have English as a first language to write research manuscripts?

A: No. If you learn college-level English, apply the rules presented here, and then find a good research mentor, it should be good enough. English was not my first language, and I did not learn great reading/writing skills until college in my career. I did not publish any manuscripts as a first author until my final year of med school, while many of my peers already had several publications when they were applying to med school.

Q: I feel like I will never learn to write research papers. Should I give up?

A: No. Writing papers is like riding a bike or seeing your first consult and writing the H/P. Your first attempt will be bad. Your work will improve. A good mentor can help your work improve faster.

Q: Do you need to have good reading/writing SAT or MCAT scores to write research manuscripts?

A: No. There is probably some baseline score/level that most people need. However, for context, mine were relatively bad (even below average on my first attempt of the MCAT) and were definitely not what got me into medical school.

Q: Do you need to enjoy reading and writing to write research manuscripts?

A: No. I don't like reading most books. As a young child, when I tried to read a book, my mind would be thinking about something else, and then I would get to the end of a page and not know what I had read. In secondary school and college, I did not do well in most English or social studies-type courses that made me read books. I have always liked books that can get to their point fast. Most books I consume today need to be in audio format, and then I play them at 1.3× while doing something else. Similarly, I write to get to the point quickly.

Q: Do I need to use this guide perfectly to publish papers? What if I do not agree with some points?
A: The rules presented in this book will apply to >95% of manuscripts you encounter. Nonetheless, this book is meant to be like scaffolding in building a house. Use the scaffolding, then remove it as needed, and make edits that you think will make your work better.

Q: What is the shortest amount of time needed to write a manuscript?
A: A few hours. If you know the prospectus already and your team can generate data to make good tables/figures, then putting this into the manuscript will take minutes. Writing results takes about 20–40 min. Writing the methods should take ~30 min, and you can ask the biostatisticians to add their blessing. The intro should take ~30 min, assuming you already know the relevant studies and can use Google to find appropriate references. The discussion can take 30–60 min. Most of the time will be spent dealing with frustrating minutiae: Why are the references not syncing? Why are the figures not saving a high-resolution version? Why is the spacing off? and so forth.

Jacksonville, FL, USA Nicholas G. Zaorsky

Contributions and Acknowledgements

The contents of the book come from my own personal experiences in writing and reviewing >1000 manuscripts; advice from colleagues, researchers, and physicians; and the references listed at the end of the book. The following colleagues helped to improve the quality of the work, listed alphabetically:

- Sam Bakhoum, MD, PhD
- Priscilla Brastianos, MD
- Mark Buyyounouski, MD (helped me write my first paper)
- Aadel Chaudhuri, MD, PhD
- Pippa Cosper, MD, PhD
- Vernon Chinchilli, PhD
- Brian Davis, MD, PhD
- Adam Dicker, MD, PhD
- Robert Den, MD, PhD
- Freddy Escorcia, MD, PhD
- Felix Feng, MD, PhD
- Gary Freedman, MD
- Stephen Freedland, MD
- Clifton David Fuller, MD
- Gianluca Giannarini, MD
- Karen Hoffman, MD
- Emma Holliday, MD
- Eric Lehrer, MD
- Alex Louie, MD
- Paul L Nguyen, MD

- Randall Kimple, MD, PhD
- Amar U Kishan, MD
- Vedang Murthy, MD
- David Palma, MD, PhD
- Joshua Palmer, MD
- Drew Ridge, MD
- Chris Sciamanna, MD, MPH
- Kathryn Schmitz, PhD
- Shankar Siva, MD, PhD
- Daniel Spratt, MD
- Corey Speers, MD
- Yilun Sun, PhD
- Leila Tchelebi, MD
- Daniel Trifiletti, MD
- Alison C Tree, MD
- Charles R Thomas, MD, PhD
- Tim Showalter, MD
- Ming Wang, PhD
- Sue Yom, MD, PhD

Meghan Keating provided editing and revision for this textbook. Meghan converted many of the parts published on Twitter/X into this readable format. Meghan also revised several of the chapters, including "Choosing a project," "Reviewing the literature," "Writing the methods," "Writing the title," "Using other programs," "How to choose a journal to submit your manuscript to," and "Publicizing your work."

Competing Interests The author has no competing interests to declare that are relevant to the content of this work.

Contents

Part I

The Project and Involved Parties

Finding a Research Mentor

1

Definition of a mentor: "an experienced and trusted advisor."

Why do you need a research mentor?

- Helps you publish research
  - Formulate a question.
  - Gather/synthesize data.
  - Write a manuscript.
- Provides guidance in your clinical training.

What are the effects of mentorship?

- Although there are no randomized trials evaluating effects of mentorship, trainees with good mentorship are usually more successful.
- Good mentorship produces trainees who:
  - Are more productive (e.g., publications, grants).
  - Attain positions and promotions more rapidly.
  - Are more likely to stay at an institution of choice.

How do I find and contact a mentor?

- Finding a mentor:
  - Word of mouth through other mentees.
  - Internet search [e.g., PubMed, Google Scholar, X (formerly Twitter)] for research you are interested in, performed by doctors at your institution.

N. G. Zaorsky, *Writing a Medical Research Manuscript*, https://doi.org/10.1007/978-3-032-20276-5_1

- Contacting a mentor:
  - Work directly in clinic, then ask about opportunities.
  - “Cold email” (i.e., without knowing mentor) about potential opportunities.

What are the qualities of a good research mentor?

- First or senior author on many works.
- Content expert.
- Determined and persistent.
- Critical of your work, but not negative:
  - Leaves many helpful comments.
  - Does not just say, “looks good. Submit.”
- Flexible to meet/message.

How do I evaluate a mentor I have not worked with?

- There is no good single metric.
- Common methods include:
  - Word of mouth.
  - Gut feeling from initial encounters.
  - Response to your email.
  - Publications with trainees as first authors.
  - Publications with trainees as coauthors.

Mentorship researchers have proposed several frameworks for evaluating mentor effectiveness. Across studies, five recurring domains emerge: communication, feedback, research guidance, career development, and psychosocial support.

How do you evaluate a mentor you have worked with?

Mentorship question domain

“My mentor …”	Meeting, communication	Expectations, feedback	Research support	Career development	Psychosocial support
Is accessible	Yes				
Is an active listener	Yes	Yes			
Has professional expertise			Yes		
Encourages me to establish independent career		Yes	Yes		
Provides useful critiques		Yes	Yes		
Motivates me to improve			Yes		
Provides guidance on professional issues				Yes	
Acknowledges my contributions		Yes		Yes	
Has interest in my career					Yes
Helps me formulate clear goals				Yes	
Builds my professional network				Yes	
Provides advice on scholarly work		Yes	Yes		
Is supportive of work-life balance					Yes
Is overall a good mentor	Yes	Yes	Yes	Yes	Yes

Adapted from: Yukawa, *PLoS ONE*, 2020; Zerzan, *Academic Med*, 2009

Diagnosing and treating mentorship malpractice

Category	Mentor Type	Core Issue	Warning Signs	Common Mentee Mistakes	Recommended Response
Active	The Hijacker	Prior failures or insecurity drive attempts to control projects and recognition.	Concern about being surpassed; excessive focus on authorship, funding, or status.	Giving away leadership roles, authorship, or ownership of ideas.	Leave the relationship promptly; these situations rarely improve.
Active	The Exploiter	Prioritizes personal goals over mentee development.	Assigns tasks that mainly benefit the mentor; expects loyalty or gratitude.	Accepting work that offers little educational or career value.	Set clear boundaries and seek independent mentorship. Exit if trust erodes.
Active	The Possessor	Fear of losing influence over the mentee.	Discourages outside mentors, collaborations, or independent opportunities.	Becoming isolated within a single mentor's network.	Build a mentoring team and openly address concerns.
Passive	The Bottleneck	Insufficient time, interest, or organizational capacity.	Delayed feedback, missed meetings, slow decisions, poor follow-through.	Waiting indefinitely for responses or approvals.	Establish deadlines, document expectations, and escalate when necessary.
Passive	The Peacemaker	Avoids conflict and prioritizes collegial relationships.	Hesitates to advocate for resources, promotions, or difficult conversations.	Assuming the mentor will champion your interests.	Develop additional mentors who can advocate more assertively.
Passive	The Celebrity	Success and external commitments limit availability.	Frequent travel, heavy speaking schedule, limited access.	Accepting minimal interaction as sufficient mentorship.	Schedule meetings well in advance and supplement with co-mentors.

Figure. Diagnosing mentorship malpractice. (Adapted from Chopra, JAMA, 2016)

What should I do before contacting a potential research mentor?

- Research the mentor:
  - Know their body of work and content expertise.
  - Does this mentor routinely work with trainees?
  - Are the trainees coauthors on PubMed articles?
  - Are the articles published in a reasonable time?
  - If possible, ask prior mentees how their experiences has been.

What should the mentee provide during initial email contact with a potential mentor?

- Name.
- Training level.
- Brief intro and background.
- Skillset: biostatistics, app creation, etc.
- Reason for email:
  - Interest in particular project vs. any project, given your background.
  - Timeframe, if applicable.
- Ask to meet formally (in person or virtually).
- Attach CV.
- Important notes:
  - Do not send an email longer than the screen of your phone.
  - Contact just one or two potential mentors initially.

What should the mentee provide during an in-person or virtual visit with a potential mentor?

- Send the mentor prep material, as needed:
  - Most recent version of manuscript, figures, and response letter.
  - Send all documents together rather than just most recent version of a table/figure.
  - Questions.
  - Roadblocks.
- Establish your involvement in the project and author line order.

What should the mentee provide after an in-person or virtual visit with a potential mentor?

- Send a thank you note.
- Summarize the meeting:
  - Next steps you will take.
  - Next steps you need from the research team.
  - Future plans to meet.
- Send updates as needed.
- If you commit to a project, finish it.
- ***Do not ghost your potential mentor.***

Which mentorship relationships succeed and which do not?

Mentoring relationships that succeed are reciprocal, involve mutual respect, have clear expectations from both parties, involve a personal connection, and have shared values.[2]

- Succeed:
  - Reciprocity.
  - Mutual respect.
  - Clear expectations.
  - Personal connection.
  - Shared values.
- ***Do not succeed:***
  - ***Poor communication.***
  - ***Lack of commitment.***
  - ***Personality differences.***
  - ***Perceived (or real) competition.***
  - ***Conflicts of interest.***
  - ***Inexperienced mentor.***

Evaluation of a mentee who is writing a medical research manuscript

Category	1 = failing	2 = below expectations	3 = at expectations	4 = exceeds expectations	5 = outstanding
Writing quality and attention to detail	Does not follow guidelines.	Major deviations from guidelines. Messy.	Good grammar, syntax, spelling. Minor deviations from guidelines.	Follows guidelines and instructions. No typos. No issues with references. Checks figures and tables. Consistent terminology.	Same, but at level of a senior author. Model or teacher for others.
Promptness	Does not reply. Ghosting.	Frequently delayed responses; unreliable communication.	Replies in 1-2 weeks.	Replies in hours-days.	Replies in hours-days, with tentative plan, even if weeks-months needed for longer response.
Receptiveness to feedback	Dismisses or ignores feedback.	Accepts it but does not incorporate it.	Incorporates it when directed.	Proactively seeks it and not discouraged by negative feedback.	Same, but at level of a senior author. Model or teacher for others.
Professionalism and teamwork	Unprofessional. The "4 Horsemen": criticism, stonewalling, defensiveness, contempt.	Occasional dismissiveness or failure to acknowledge co-authors' contributions.	Respectful, compassionate, kind, collaborative.	Same, but more emotionally mature.	Same, but at level of a senior author. Model or teacher for others.
Intellectual engagement and initiative	Disengaged or inattentive.	Some missed meetings and limited engagement.	Attends all meetings and engages in discussion.	Independently identifies solutions, contributes thoughtful questions/ideas, anticipates next steps, shows curiosity.	Same, but at level of a senior author. Model or teacher for others.
Dress code and appearance	Camera off, or underdressed.	Sometimes inattentive or unprepared presentation.	Camera on. Dressed appropriately.	Consistently well-presented; professional appearance in all settings.	Formal attire in person.
Technical research skills, unique abilities	Requires substantial remediation.	Limited ability to independently perform research tasks.	Solid understanding of basic tools (MS Office, statistics).	Programming, biostats, app creation, illustration, AI, social media creation, etc.	Model or teacher for others in these areas.
Research ethics and integrity	Fabrication, falsification, misrepresentation.	Minor deviations.	Follows policies on responsible conduct of research, data management, institutional review board practices, conflicts of interest, authorship.	Proactively identifies potential ethical issues.	Model or teacher for others in these areas.
Grit, drive, independent growth trajectory	Declining performance despite available resources and mentorship.	Requires significant external support and repeated prompting to make progress; limited self-direction.	Needs minor prompting.	Performing at a high level in a context-specific manner. Overall positive career trajectory.	Overcame substantial obstacles to excel in these areas.

Advice for Mentees

2

Keys to Maximizing Academic Productivity as a Trainee

Find the right mentor/senior author

- The mentor is arguably the most important part of the publishing puzzle. Good mentorship for a project is more important than the topic of the project. Research this person, know their body of work, if they work with trainees. Ask former trainees about the mentor.
- Characteristics of a good mentor:
  - Content expert with productive publication history, especially recently.
  - Senior author on many works, trainees as first authors.
  - Determined and persistent.
  - Critical of your work but not negative.
  - Flexible to meet and message.
  - Not "mentor malpractice": not a hijacker, exploiter, possessor, bottleneck, country clubber, world traveler. Not a shark.
- You need people you can trust to tell you the truth. You need radical candor—someone who cares personally but also challenges you directly. Your mentors should be "door openers," invested in exposing you to opportunities for your long-term career success.

N. G. Zaorsky, *Writing a Medical Research Manuscript*,
https://doi.org/10.1007/978-3-032-20276-5_2

- As we get older, we start to get conflicting advice from different mentors. Sometimes, the advice is also in contrast to what our close friends and family recommend. Ultimately, you have to decide which pieces of advice are best.
- Collaborate nationally and internationally. In 2025, it is rare to have high impact projects from a single department in one institution.

Find the right project

- Have a prospectus for each project:
  - Background: 1–2 paragraphs of the issue in medicine, what this project is planning to solve. Then a purpose, hypothesis, aim.
  - Methods: A few sentences how data will be obtained (e.g., coding patient charts vs database). Who is the biostatistician who can help? What are the planned journal(s) for submission (if applicable)?
  - Author line, where the trainee will be.
  - Project timeline. Will this be completed by the time you move to the next career stage?
- Types of projects with highest success rates:

  Retrospective case series with data already available (e.g., national database). Why?

  1, no protected health info, usually no or minimal IRB requirement.

  2, data already collected.

  3, no recoding of data.

  4, can copy methods from other studies PRN.

  5, large databases are available for many diseases, patient cohort types.

  Systematic review +/– meta-analysis. Why?

  1, you can find niche topic in almost any area.

  2, study-level data already collected.

  3, no protected health info, no IRB.

  4, data are yours.

  5, work on your own time, at any place.

  6, easy for follow-up works.

  7, cookie cutter methods.

- Projects with lower success rates:
  - Case series from your home institution/"Freedom from everything": you code many variables and outcomes for patients in the hospital, without a clear purpose. If you are presented with a potential project where you have to code 100 variables per patient without a clear purpose, you may be better off avoiding the project.
  - Most case reports.
- Minimize regulatory burden: institutional review boards, data use agreements, etc.
- Use your skill set (e.g., biostatistics, writing, knowledge of field).
- Don't take on more than you can handle. Finish your projects. Take on new projects carefully. Balance your projects with the rest of your life.

Communicate effectively with your team

- Send short emails with key points, all relevant files (e.g., manuscript, figures, tables, disclosure forms), timeline, next steps, question you are asking.
  - Don't send an email longer than the screen of your phone. Consider asking to meet and discuss further—sometimes, it is faster to discuss on the phone, via zoom, or in person instead of typing it out.
- If you ask for a meeting, be clear why.
  - A few days before the meeting, send the most recent version of all relevant files, i.e., manuscript, figures, response letter questions, roadblocks.
  - Make sure your meeting has a purpose. Faculty members have limited time and are asked to attend many meetings. Be sure to consider:

    Is this meeting an appropriate length (i.e., can it be 30 min instead of 60?)

    Could the content of this meeting have been sent in a PDF? Could the PDF have been an email?
- Underpromise and overdeliver. For example, say you will send the results in 2 weeks and then send the full paper in 1 week.

- Respond to emails within 1–2 weeks max. You can also reply within a few days to say "I am working on this and will get back to you by X."
- At all times, be able to describe the prospectus of your project, including background, purpose, general methods, and your individual role. Your prospectus is fair game for interviews and will hopefully materialize into a publication.
- Establish your involvement in the project and author line order early.
  - If you do the bulk of writing, you could be the first author.
  - If you have a more peripheral role, you could be a coauthor.
  - Advocate for yourself. Authorship can be seen as a recognition of your contribution to the work, so if you have had meaningful involvement in the project, you should discuss authorship with your mentor.
  - Update coauthors PRN (e.g., submissions, revisions).
- Don't ghost your mentor. Mentors can't read your mind: If something has changed, if you don't have interest in the project, if you are sick or have a family emergency, just say so. A good mentor shouldn't be offended.
  - If changing institutions (e.g., graduation), provide your new contact info ASAP.
- Treat your manuscript like your baby. You should know everything about it: the status, what needs to be done. You are responsible for catching all grammar/syntax errors, typos, formatting issues.

	overall direction of project	**writing**	**checking grammar, syntax, formatting**	**providing methodological or content expertise**
senior author	primary job	secondary job	secondary job	primary job
coauthor w content expertise			secondary job	primary job
coauthor who is a trainee		secondary job	primary job	
first author		primary job	primary job	

Figure. Authors and their roles in manuscript writing

Optimize your writing environment and time

- Learn how to write a medical research manuscript, e.g., use this guide.🙂
- At least dual monitors, 1440p.

  - With a dual screen monitor and the Split Window tool, you can have your manuscript, response letter, reference manager, PDFs, and browser all open at once.
- No distractions like social media.
- Use referencing software (e.g., EndNote, Zotero). Do not reference manually, it is not worth your time.
- Edit PowerPoint registry for high resolution images.
- Use your designated academic time to do research.
- Make a designated writing time each week. Write at least 3 days per week (like going to the gym).

Keep the momentum

- Don't put off until tomorrow what you can do today. Examples: writing, submission, revision, sending emails. Do these within 1–2 weeks max.
- The longer a project takes, the longer it will take. This is also the intern adage: The more time you spend working in the hospital, the more time you will spend working in the hospital.
- Done is better than perfect. Perfect is the enemy of good. Give yourself a deadline and write what you can. Once you have a draft, send it to your mentor.
- Keep the paper submitted, in some journal.
- Keep a live list of all ongoing projects, with coauthors, status, what needs to be done.
- Check in with your mentor every ~2–4 weeks PRN: "Did we hear back from the biostatistician? What should I do next?"
- Check in with the journal after >1–2 months PRN: "Can you please send an update on the submission?"
- Success is going from failure to failure without losing enthusiasm. Do not be discouraged with rejection. Move on to the next journal. Submitted projects are typically rejected multiple times before being accepted. "Batting 300" in academia is excellent.
- Finish your projects, i.e., get them to be a manuscript. Abstracts and unfinished works have limited value.
- Take on new projects carefully, balance them with your life.
- Ask your mentorship board of trustees for advice.

General Advice for Medical School

Attitude is everything

- Be nice, hardworking, and smart. And in that order.
  - You don't have to be the brightest light bulb; just shine as bright as you can all the time. Do your best.
  - Ten things that require 0 talent: being on time, work ethic, effort, body language, energy, attitude, passion, being coachable, doing extra, being prepared.
  - Three, As to success: affability, availability, and ability.
  - "It is better to remain silent and be thought a fool than to speak and to remove all doubt."
- Be a multiplier, not a diminisher.

Take every opportunity as one to learn

- Being in medical school is a privilege. Don't forget why you went into medical school to be a physician. Medical school is like training for a triathlon. Being outside of your comfort zone, feeling the burn, is necessary for success. When weightlifters go to the gym, they go with other weightlifters; i.e., they are all there to put in the work together so they can see results. Successful medical students do the same.
- You are the average of the five people you spend the most time with. Spend your time with people you can learn from.
- Adapt a mindset of understanding first, and then committing information to memory.
- Success consists of going from failure to failure without loss of enthusiasm.
- There are at least two problems with medicine: (1) in 100 years, half of it will be proven to be false; (2) we don't know which half.
- Seek feedback proactively and often: "What are the expectations of me?" "Am I meeting them?"
- Hold questions until the end, read the room, and ask if there is a good time.

Be professional

- "A reputation takes decades to build and minutes to destroy."

- Always speak well of people. Others remember when you speak well of someone; if you speak poorly of someone, they wonder: what do they say about me behind my back?
- Be promiscuous with your positive emotions: tell people what makes them great, what they are doing well, what you are enjoying. The biggest wasted resource in the world is positive thoughts because most of them are not articulated.
  - Bring positive energy. Negativity multiplies and smiles are infectious.
  - Compliment people when they do a good job.
  - Be a good teammate. Support your fellow trainees and don't flex on them.
- "You can easily judge the character of a person by how they treat those who can do nothing for them."
- Read the room and match the energy. "It is better to be unmemorable than to be remembered for a bad reason."
- Be professional in all locations: in school; in public: at the bar, at the baseball game, at the neighborhood party, etc; on especially on social media because it is permanent.
- Dress professionally:
  - "What you wear is how you present yourself to the world. Fashion is language."
  - "Dressing well is a form of good manners."
- Assume all emails will later be read publicly. Do not send scathing emails and be wary of those who do.

Take care of yourself

- Our life is: 1/3 work, 1/3 family and friends, 1/3 sleep. Imbalance in any third will negatively affect the other parts. After work, you should feel like you can't wait to go spend time with your friends and family. After time at home with family, you should feel like you can't wait to get to bed. After a good sleep, you should feel like you can't wait to get to work.
  - Practice good diet, exercise, and sleep.
  - "Sleep is the single most effective thing we can do to reset our brain and body health each day"—*Matthew Walker, Why We Sleep*.
  - Take sick and personal days when needed.

- Recognize your work efficiency curve. You may be able to work or study at 100% for 4 h, then 80% for 2 h, and then <20% for the remaining time.

Approach research projects with discretion

- Research is a complement to, but not a replacement for, clinical skills.
- Good mentorship for a project is more important than the topic of the project.
- Abstracts have much less value than published manuscripts. A series of abstracts with no conversion to manuscripts may be detrimental.

Build a mentorship team

- You need people you can trust to tell you the truth. You need radical candor—someone who cares personally but also challenges you directly. Your mentors should be "door openers," invested in exposing you to opportunities for your long-term career success.
- Consider:
  - Physicians in your specialty of interest, physicians outside of your specialty of interest.
  - Residents.
  - Other students.
  - Significant other.

Stay organized

- Keep a professional folder. Diplomas, BLS, ACLS, certificates, transcripts, licenses, DEA license, medical license, clearance, flu shots, evaluations, letters of recommendation, published articles, awards, "small wins," etc.
- The best time to update your professional catalog (e.g., CV) is often on downtime during a trip.
- Use a calendar to keep track of assignments, exam, deadlines, blocks, interviews, etc.
- Set deadlines for yourself.
- Keep a clean email inbox. Consider using your unread email as a to do list.

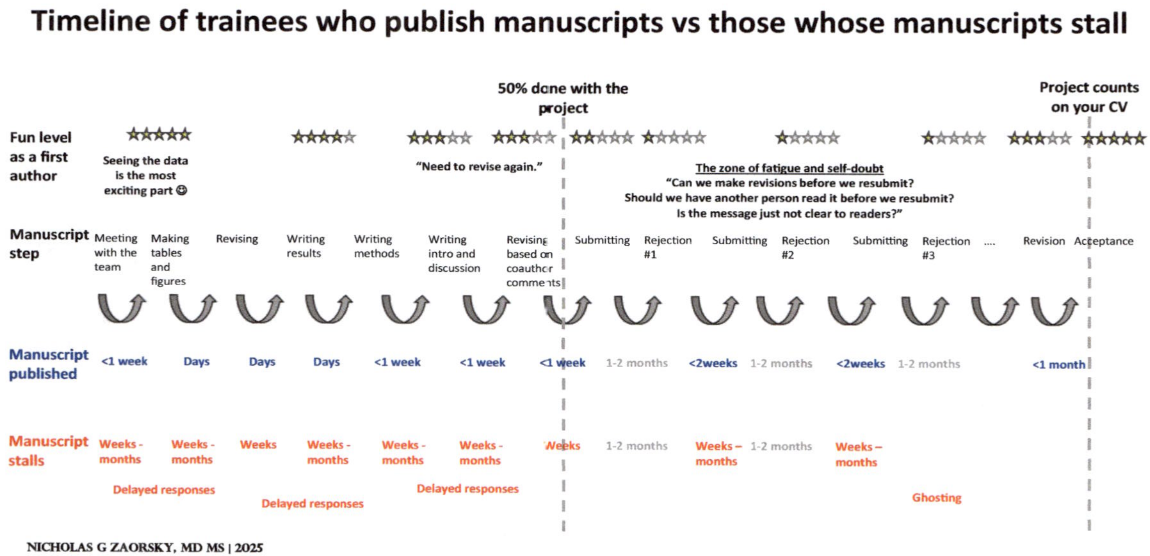

Figure. Spectrum of authors who succeed in publishing (blue) vs those who fail (red) over the manuscript writing process. These types of authors are not mutually exclusive; an author can move from being successful to unsuccessful and vice versa during their career, and while writing each manuscript. The most exciting parts of publishing are seeing the initial data, making tables and figures to tell the narrative, and then having the manuscript published. Parts in the middle of these two milestones have variable levels of fun and are sometimes onerous, boring, and busywork. Having the manuscript written is oftentimes only 50% through the entire process, and arguably, the parts before this are more fun than those after it (e.g., seeing rejections, revising and resubmitting). An author who can quickly move from one step to the next will have the greatest success in publishing. Both types of authors will be limited by the manuscript submission and review process

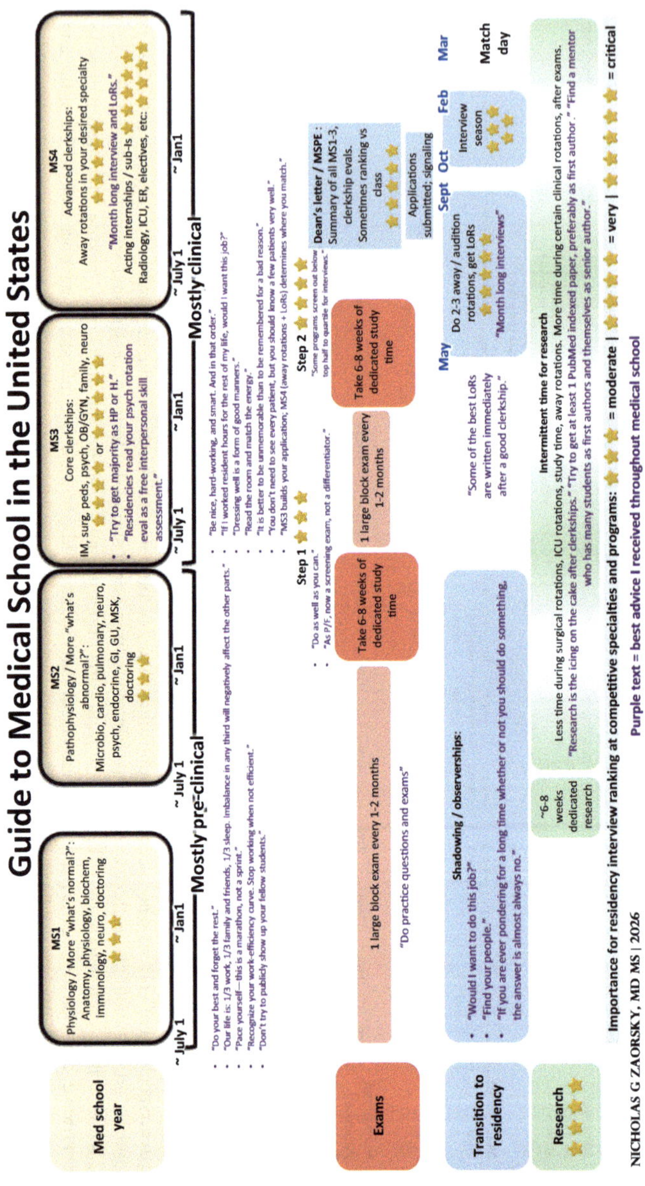
Guide to Medical School in the United States
Med school year
MS1
Physiology / More "what's normal?":
Anatomy, physiology, biochem, immunology, neuro, doctoring
MS2
Pathophysiology / More "what's abnormal?":
Microbio, cardio, pulmonary, neuro, psych, endocrine, GI, GU, MSK, doctoring
MS3
Core clerkships:
IM, surg, peds, psych, OB/GYN, family, neuro
or
"Try to get majority as HP or H."
"Residencies read your psych rotation eval as a free interpersonal skill assessment."
MS4
Advanced clerkships:
Away rotations in your desired specialty
"Month long interview and LoRs."
Acting internships / sub-Is
Radiology, ICU, ER, electives, etc:
~ July 1
~ Jan1
~ July 1
~ Jan1
~ July 1
~ Jan1
~ July 1
~ Jan1
Mostly pre-clinical
Mostly clinical
"Do your best and forget the rest."
"Our life is: 1/3 work, 1/3 family and friends, 1/3 sleep. Imbalance in any third will negatively affect the other parts."
"Pace yourself—this is a marathon, not a sprint."
"Recognize your work-efficiency curve. Stop working when not efficient."
"Don't try to publicly show up your fellow students."
"Be nice, hard-working, and smart. And in that order."
"If I worked resident hours for the rest of my life, would I want this job?"
"Dressing well is a form of good manners."
"Read the room and match the energy."
"It is better to be unmemorable than to be remembered for a bad reason."
"You don't need to see every patient, but you should know a few patients very well."
"MS3 builds your application; MS4 (away rotations + LoRs) determines where you match."
Step 1
"Do as well as you can."
"As P/F, now a screening exam, not a differentiator."
Step 2
"Some programs screen out below top half to quartile for interviews."
Dean's letter / MSPE : Summary of all MS1-3, clerkship evals. Sometimes ranking vs class
Exams
1 large block exam every 1-2 months
"Do practice questions and exams"
Take 6-8 weeks of dedicated study time
1 large block exam every 1-2 months
Take 6-8 weeks of dedicated study time
Applications submitted; signaling
May
Sept
Oct
Feb
Mar
Transition to residency
Shadowing / observerships:
"Would I want to do this job?"
"Find your people."
"If you are ever pondering for a long time whether or not you should do something, the answer is almost always no."
"Some of the best LoRs are written immediately after a good clerkship."
Do 2-3 away / audition rotations, get LoRs
"Month long interviews"
Interview season
Match day
Research
~6-8 weeks dedicated research
Intermittent time for research
Less time during surgical rotations, ICU rotations, study time, away rotations. More time during certain clinical rotations, after exams.
"Research is the icing on the cake after clerkships." "Try to get at least 1 PubMed indexed paper, preferably as first author." "Find a mentor who has many students as first authors and themselves as senior author."
Importance for residency interview ranking at competitive specialties and programs: = moderate | = very | = critical
NICHOLAS G ZAORSKY, MD MS | 2026
Purple text = best advice I received throughout medical school

Advice for Mentors

3

- Understand the skills, goals, and timeline of your mentee. Align these to a particular project. What does the mentee want for the next stage of their career?

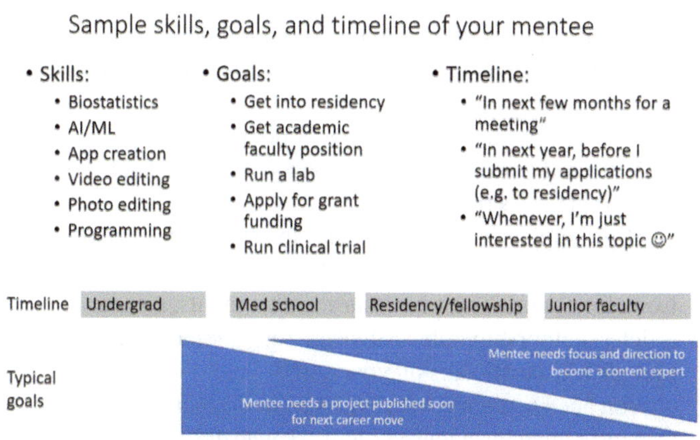

Figure. Comparing skills and goals of mentees on a timeline

- Present your project idea (i.e., prospectus) to a larger audience before getting the mentee involved. Your goal is to get the project to a PubMed publication. If it's not published, it's not as helpful for your mentee.

N. G. Zaorsky, *Writing a Medical Research Manuscript*,
https://doi.org/10.1007/978-3-032-20276-5_3

- Get revisions back within a few weeks. (You asked your mentee to do the same.)
  - If you tell your mentee to make edits, and then make more edits, and then more, try not to go full circle to the original version.
- Avoid the scenario in a project where your mentee has to go back through all of the patient charts and pull data for a new variable.
- Provide constructive feedback with lots of comments.
  - It is great to see tracked changes, thoughts, references, etc.
  - The language in our papers is revised considerably by all authors, and our work improves as a result.
- Don't scut out your mentee. Some jobs are necessary for the success of the project, but other jobs create busy work and won't lead to publication in the mentee's time window.
- Don't ghost your mentee. (You ask the same of your mentee.)
- Encourage collaboration nationally and internationally.
  - Projects that are based out of a single institution are rarely high impact and will bounce among journals.
  - Help your mentee get connected with international content experts, especially as they progress in their career.
- Aim for a high impact project and journal.
  - You want a project that will change the field, published in a journal that is read broadly.
  - High impact projects can land in reputable journals. Low impact projects will have trouble getting into any journal.
- Look for opportunities for your mentee: grants, awards, review articles, authorship, jobs. Advocate for your mentee.
- Include biostatisticians on your author line.
  - You need someone with expertise in the methods.
  - Most high impact journals will ask who did your biostatistics. If it was a trainee, prepare for rejection.
  - Avoiding contractual relationships will provide more consistent results and will help build long-term relationships that can result in numerous successful projects.
- Try to assign one mentee to one project. If you assign 2+ mentees to one project without understanding their unique skills and collaboration potential, it can get confusing. One person will end up doing most of the work.

- Avoid mentorship malpractice.
  - Don't take hostage a mentee's ideas or projects and label them as your own.
  - Don't drag down your mentee with low-yield activities. Be invested in fostering meaningful growth.
  - Don't dominate your mentee. Don't disparage mentees, or discourage them from reaching out to others.
  - Don't take on mentees if you don't have the bandwidth or the desire to do so.
  - Don't avoid conflict. Having difficult but necessary conversations will benefit your mentee far more than being "the nice guy."
  - Be aware of your other commitments. If you are extremely busy with meetings, speaking engagements, and leadership positions, your mentee may be at risk of being left behind.
- Create a list/calendar of conferences with submission deadlines for research projects. Tell your team about the deadline many months in advance.
- When the time is right, share your data with an international team working on the same question. Manuscripts are often rejected, because it is a single institution and limited data set. If you join a larger group, the work will go farther.
- Start a manuscript review group with your colleagues, department, trainees, etc. People will provide comments on your work and it will improve. Their works will improve by reading your research. Everyone wins.
- If you want to write an authoritative high impact review article, then contact international leaders on this topic, compose a synopsis, and mail it to the editor in chief of a journal.

Evaluation of a mentee who is writing a medical research manuscript

NICHOLAS G ZAORSKY, MD MS | 2026

Adapted from the textbook: Zaorsky NG. *Writing a Medical Research Manuscript*. Springer Nature Switzerland; 2026. ISBN: 9783032202758.

Category	1 = failing	2 = below expectations	3 = at expectations	4 = exceeds expectations	5 = outstanding
Writing quality and attention to detail	Does not follow guidelines.	Major deviations from guidelines. Messy.	Good grammar, syntax, spelling. Minor deviations from guidelines.	Follows guidelines and instructions. No typos. No issues with references. Checks figures and tables. Consistent terminology.	Same, but at level of a senior author. Model or teacher for others.
Promptness	Does not reply. Ghosting.	Frequently delayed responses; unreliable communication.	Replies in 1-2 weeks.	Replies in hours-days.	Replies in hours-days, with tentative plan, even if weeks-months needed for longer response.
Receptiveness to feedback	Dismisses or ignores feedback.	Accepts it but does not incorporate it.	Incorporates it when directed.	Proactively seeks it and not discouraged by negative feedback.	Same, but at level of a senior author. Model or teacher for others.
Professionalism and teamwork	Unprofessional. The "4 Horsemen": criticism, stonewalling, defensiveness, contempt.	Occasional dismissiveness or failure to acknowledge co-authors' contributions.	Respectful, compassionate, kind, collaborative.	Same, but more emotionally mature.	Same, but at level of a senior author. Model or teacher for others.
Intellectual engagement and initiative	Disengaged or inattentive.	Some missed meetings and limited engagement.	Attends all meetings and engages in discussion.	Independently identifies solutions, contributes thoughtful questions/ideas, anticipates next steps, shows curiosity.	Same, but at level of a senior author. Model or teacher for others.
Dress code and appearance	Camera off or not present, or very underdressed.	Camera sometimes off, somewhat underdressed.	Camera on. Dressed appropriately.	Consistently well-presented; professional appearance in all settings.	Formal attire in person.
Technical research skills, unique abilities	Requires substantial remediation.	Limited ability to independently perform research tasks.	Solid understanding of basic tools (MS Office, statistics).	Programming, biostats, app creation, illustration, AI, social media creation, etc.	Model or teacher for others in these areas.
Research ethics and integrity	Fabrication, falsification, misrepresentation.	Minor deviations.	Follows policies on responsible conduct of research, data management, institutional review board practices, conflicts of interest, authorship.	Proactively identifies potential ethical issues.	Model or teacher for others in these areas.
Grit, drive, independent growth trajectory	Declining performance despite available resources and mentorship.	Requires significant external support and repeated prompting to make progress; limited self-direction.	Needs minor prompting.	Performing at a high level in a context-specific manner. Overall positive career trajectory.	Overcame substantial obstacles to excel in these areas.

4 Writing a Prospectus

- A prospectus/synopsis is a preliminary printed statement describes:
  - Author line.
  - Background.
  - Hypothesis/purpose.
  - Methods.
  - Where the paper will be published.
- Every paper is built around one primary research question, one hypothesis, and one central contribution.
- Avoid questions like "I must have treated 100 patients like this at the hospital. Can you find out how they did?"
- The mentor should create a prospectus/synopsis and circulate it to a core group of knowledgeable authors before proceeding.
- Most works will stop at this stage.
- Acknowledging your idea is not the best and cutting losses early is key. You will find another project. It is not worth your time to pursue a bad idea.

N. G. Zaorsky, *Writing a Medical Research Manuscript*,
https://doi.org/10.1007/978-3-032-20276-5_4

Authorship

5

- Coauthors are the equivalent of "consultants" for a patient. They can include statisticians, trainees, data collectors, topic experts, department chairs, and individuals who review/comment on your manuscript.
- Mentors should not blindly advocate for coauthors for collegiality or because "they refer patients to us." Similarly, a department chair should not be coauthor unless they contributed to the project.
- Be generous with your author lines. Include statisticians and trainees.
- When possible, summarize authorship expectations in a brief follow-up email after initial project discussions.
- Authorship is a combination of four factors:
  - Conception or design of the work; or the acquisition, analysis, or interpretation of data.
  - Drafting the work or revision.
  - Final approval.
  - Agreement to be accountable for work.

N. G. Zaorsky, *Writing a Medical Research Manuscript*,
https://doi.org/10.1007/978-3-032-20276-5_5

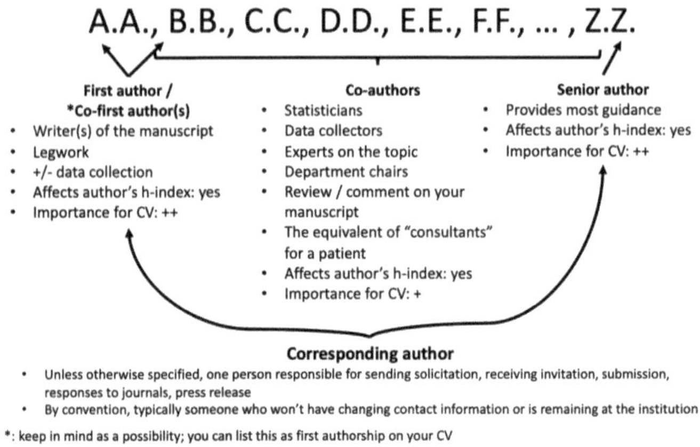

Figure. Authors and their roles

Why authorship conflicts occur?

Authorship conflicts rarely arise from a single event. They usually result from:

- Unclear expectations early in the project.
- Changes in contribution over time.
- Power differentials between trainees and senior authors.
- Poor communication or delays.
- Misalignment between academic incentives and actual work performed.

These conflicts are common, predictable, and preventable.

Best strategy: prevent conflicts early

- The most effective way to manage authorship conflict is to prevent it.
- At the start of the project, clarify:
  - Author line order.
  - Who is first author?
  - Who is senior author?
- Who are anticipated middle authors?
  - Expected contributions.

  - Who is responsible for data collection?
  - Who writes the first draft?
  - Who handles revisions and submission?
- Timeline
  - Is this feasible within the trainee's remaining time at the institution?
- Contingencies
  - What happens if a trainee leaves the institution?
  - What happens if someone contributes less or more than expected?

These discussions do not need to be formal or confrontational. A short email summary after an initial meeting is often sufficient.

Common authorship conflict scenarios and how to handle them

1. A senior author adds new authors late in the process
   - Ask (politely) what role each added author played.
   - If their contribution meets authorship criteria, accept it.
   - If not, suggest acknowledgment instead.
   - Focus on publication success, not "winning" the argument.
2. Disagreement about first authorship
   - Reframe the discussion around contribution, not seniority.
   - If contributions changed over time, reassess authorship honestly.
   - If unresolved, ask a neutral third party (e.g., another mentor) for input.
3. Mentor stops responding or delays indefinitely
   - Send a short, respectful follow-up summarizing:
     - Current status
     - What you are waiting on
     - A proposed next step
   - If delays persist and publication is at risk, ask whether it is appropriate to:
     - Submit to a lower-tier journal
     - Bring in an additional senior author
     - Transfer leadership of the project

4. Data or manuscript is "held hostage" when a trainee leaves
   - This is why authorship and data access should be clarified early.
   - If the project was your primary work, you should retain access to:
     Data
     Manuscript drafts
   - Most institutions and journals support trainee authorship continuity after graduation.

5. You did substantial work but are offered middle authorship
   - Advocate for yourself respectfully.
   - State your contributions clearly and factually.
   - Ask how authorship was determined.
   - If the answer is unsatisfactory, use this information to guide future mentor selection.

When to escalate authorship disputes?
Escalation should be rare but appropriate when:
- Your work is misrepresented.
- You are excluded after substantial contribution.
- Ethical standards are violated.

Potential escalation paths:
- Trusted senior mentor.
- Program director or division chief.
- Institutional research office (last resort).

Avoid public confrontation or emotional emails. Assume all correspondence may be reviewed later.

Key principles to remember
- Authorship reflects contribution, not rank.
- Most conflicts are due to miscommunication, not malice.
- Publishing the paper is usually more valuable than "winning" the dispute.
- Patterns matter: one conflict may be situational; repeated conflicts suggest a poor mentorship fit.

6 Choosing a Project

Choose a type of project that best fits your goals and timeframe. For medical students and residents, retrospective case series and review articles are the easiest to do.

Table: Advantages and disadvantages of various projects.

Study design	Time	Advantages	Disadvantages
Prospective trial	>5 years	• Gold standard of evidence-based medicine	• Typically not possible as a trainee
Basic science	>6 months	• Translational research possible	• Takes years • Trainee rarely primary or secondary author
Retrospective case series	1–5 months	• Can be done at most institutions • Excellent when database already present • Can combine multiple case reports	• Usually need >20–50 patients • All patients need same data • Usually needs stats

(continued)

N. G. Zaorsky, *Writing a Medical Research Manuscript*,
https://doi.org/10.1007/978-3-032-20276-5_6

Table: (continued)

Study design	Time	Advantages	Disadvantages
Review article: includes narrative review, systematic review +/− meta-analysis (see figure below for comparison)		• Can be done anywhere • Can combine multiple cases • If done well, can be accepted to high-impact journals	• Need to know subject/literature • Invited > Uninvited • Solicited > Unsolicited • Requires a comprehensive understanding of all available literature • Data extraction/data cleaning can be time consuming • Meta-analyses require stats
Survey	<3 months	• Relatively easy if high impact topic	• Need to find email addresses • Single time point • Limited by low response rates • Usually limited to low tier journals
Case report		• Easy to find • Improve by adding more cases, basic science	• Rarely accepted, especially to high impact factor journal
Commentaries			• Often commissioned by the journal, so may be difficult for mentees to publish

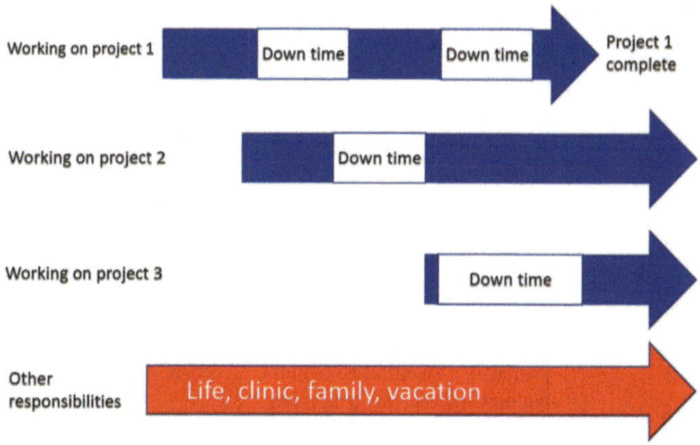

Figure. Balancing multiple projects and life responsibilities

Table: Narrative reviews vs. systematic literature reviews vs. meta-analyses

Review type	Overview	Example
Narrative review	• Overview of literature on a topic that docs not require the same strict methodological requirements as a systematic review. Is not considered comprehensive. • Serves to summarize the literature and is often used to identify areas for further research.	"This review discusses the current knowledge of metastatic cancer, including epidemiology, risk factors for death, and treatment options available."
Systematic literature of review	• Require rigorous search methodologies (specific eligibility criteria) for literature on a particular topic, e.g., Using PICOS and PRISMA. • Summarizes the literature and makes conclusions in a qualitative manner only.	"This review summarizes all randomized controlled trials of stereotactic body radiation therapy for the treatment of metastatic disease."

(continued)

Table: (continued)

Review type	Overview	Example
Meta-analysis	• Requires same degree of methodological rigor as a systematic literature review. • Involves extraction of data from included studies for statistical analysis. An outcome of interest is identified and is the focus for the paper. Sometimes secondary outcomes of interest are included. • Literature is summarized in primarily a quantitative manner, but may include some narrative results. • Can be limited by heterogeneity of available data.	"This meta-analysis evaluates 1 year local control after stereotactic body radiation therapy for oligometastatic cancer. Secondary outcomes analyzed include 1 year survival and metastatic progression."

Table: Ranking research project endeavors

Rank	Good mentor	Mentee interested in project	Data readily available
1	Yes	Yes	Yes
2	Yes	Possibly	Yes
3	Yes	Possibly	No, but obtainable
4	No	Yes	No, but obtainable
5	No	No	Yes or no

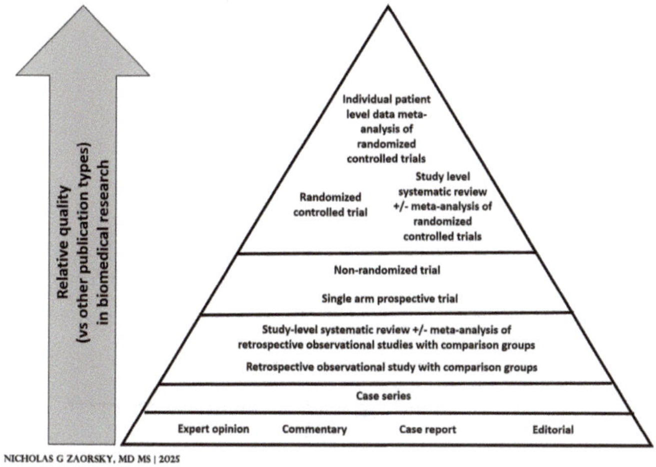

Figure. Relative quality of various types of research projects. This is a modified evidence-based research pyramid, another version is in Golden and Bass (2013). Quality of research design increases from bottom to top of pyramid. Quantity of research design in the published literature decreased from bottom to top of pyramid. Note that study-level systematic reviews of retrospective data would be of similar quality as observational studies (i.e., "garbage in = garbage out"). In contrast, patient-level data meta analysis of randomized trials can be of higher evidence than single randomized trials

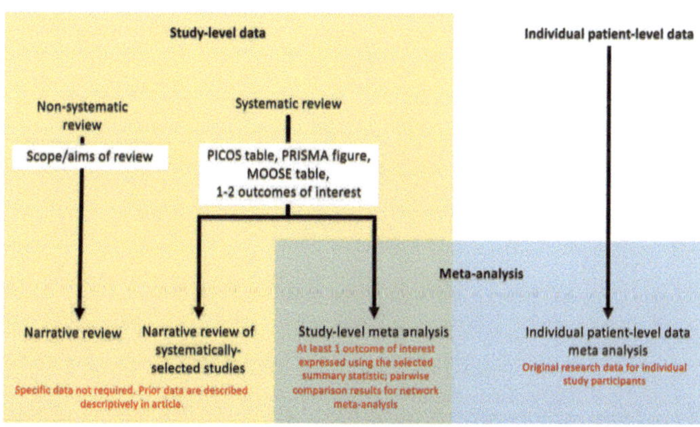

Figure. Types of review articles and meta-analyses, adapted from Lehrer et al.

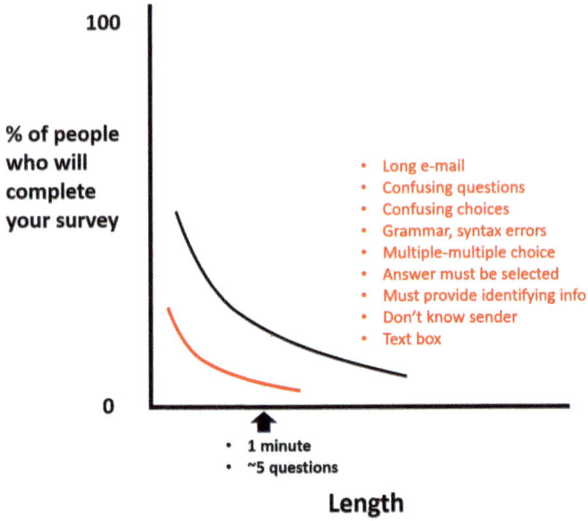

Figure. Survey research response rates and factors affecting responses

Part II

The Manuscript

7 An Overview of the Manuscript

Your manuscript should flow naturally, describing your aims, the methods you designed to reach the aims, and your findings. A good framework is as follows:

Italics = your aim or expectation

Bold = your finding or observation

Bold italics = info that gets you from the aim to the observation

Abstract
- *Purpose*.
- ***Methods***.
- ***Results***.
- **Conclusion**.

Manuscript
- *Intro to last paragraph*.
- ***Methods***.
- ***Results, tables, figures***.
- Discussion
  - **First paragraph**.
  - Ways that your findings fit into and add to current knowledge.
- **Conclusion**

N. G. Zaorsky, *Writing a Medical Research Manuscript*, https://doi.org/10.1007/978-3-032-20276-5_7

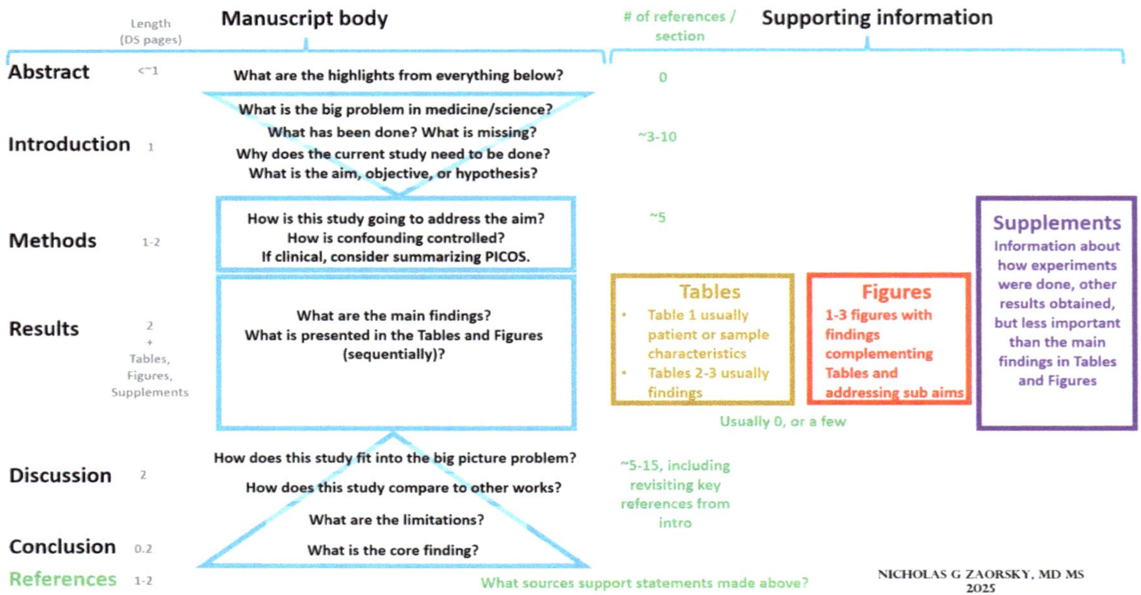

Figure. Overview and structure of a medical research manuscript. The inverted triangle represents the introduction's narrowing of ideas from general to specific. General advice: (1) tell them what you are going to say; (2) say it; and (3) tell them what you said

Writing a paper is like writing a haiku

Title/Author page	
Abstract:	~300 words, depends on journal
Intro:	1 page
Methods:	2 pages, can have supplements
Results:	2 pages, can have supplements
Discussion:	2 pages max
Conclusion:	3–5 sentences
References	
Tables	
Figure legends	

Reviewing the Literature

8

When to review the literature?

- Research mentors should have a strong understanding of the literature and include relevant contexts when creating the prospectus.
- Mentees should review the available literature after receiving the prospectus and before beginning the project.
  - Remember: you should be able to articulate the goals, design, purpose, and contexts for your project at all times.

Goal of reviewing the literature

- To understand the precedent for and contexts of your research project. More simply, to identify what is known and not known about the topic, and to formulate the purpose of your paper accordingly.

How to review the literature?

- Based on your research question and study goals, create a list of key terms relevant to your topic. Refine and add to this list as needed.
- Use a research-specific search tool, i.e., Google Scholar or PubMed.
  - Google Scholar will find literature and sort it based on a combination of date of publications, citations, access. Scholar will also link to researchers who have created profiles online and link to their research. Example: your paper is on metastatic cancer:

N. G. Zaorsky, *Writing a Medical Research Manuscript*,
https://doi.org/10.1007/978-3-032-20276-5_8

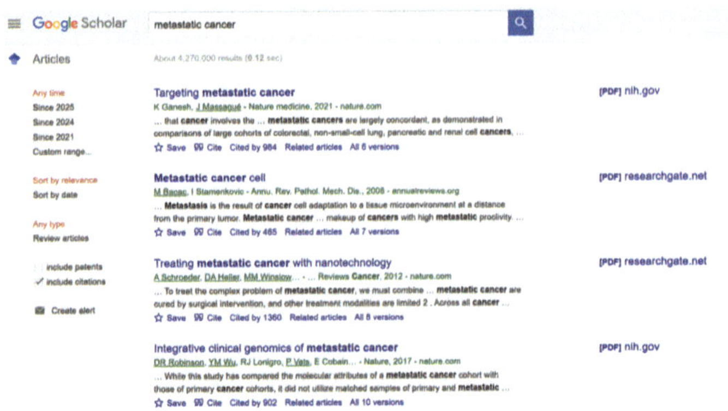

Figure. Searching on google scholar

  - PubMed is also a good option, but doesn't sort by relevance as well.
    With PubMed, you can search using MeSH terms, a set of key terms which are organized categorically to help identify literature relevant to a topic
    To assist with identifying MeSH terms, you can use the MeSH on Demand Tool: https://meshb.nlm.nih.gov/MeSHonDemand
- Use Boolean operators such as [AND], [OR], and [NOT] to refine your search terms.
- Use wildcard searches to include similar search terms
  - *(asterisk) replaces a string of characters: i.e., metasta* = metastasis, metastatic, etc.
  - ? (question mark) replaces a single character: i.e., cancer* = cancer, cancers, etc.
- Use AI programs like OpenEvidence, ChatGPT, Claude, etc. Ask them to help find relevant references by evaluating your proposal and searching current guidelines.
- Cross-check references
  - Use the references of the papers you identify to help find additional relevant works you may have missed in your search.
- Ask a librarian for help
  - If you are affiliated with an academic institution, chances are you have dedicated research librarians who are experts in literature searches.

- Stay organized
  - Organize your citations using a citation manager like EndNote or Zotero.
  - When performing a literature review, it can be helpful to summarize key aspects of papers in a document to make them easier to reference later. (You can also use the notes function in Zotero to do this).

9 Writing the Results

Results Text

The results section is one of the most important parts of the research manuscript, telling readers what the study found, without providing background or interpretation. Your results section (including tables and figures) will be the first part of the paper you write. This is one of the first parts of the paper that reviewers read. If this part is not clear, they will reject your paper.

When to write?

- After you make the tables and figures.

Goal of this section

- To summarize broad themes of your data, including all tables, figures, supplements.
- To NOT interpret the data.

Format

- Length: ~2 double spaced pages, 11–12 point font for most full text manuscripts. Should be longer than the discussion section, usually.
- Succinctly, use numbers and statistical tests to report findings.
- Consistency in significant figures is important; rarely are >3–4 sig figs needed.

N. G. Zaorsky, *Writing a Medical Research Manuscript*,
https://doi.org/10.1007/978-3-032-20276-5_9

- Be quantitative: list specific estimates, CIs, p-values, HRs, ORs, RRs
  - *Whenever possible, report CIs alongside point estimates to convey precision.*
- Reference all tables, figures, and supplements.
- Report the **relative risk** and the **absolute risk**.
  - Always report both when possible.
  - Also report absolute event rates whenever feasible.
  - If appropriate, calculate number needed to treat or harm (NNT) or (NNH).
  - Reserve interpretation for the discussion but do not hide magnitude.
  - **Relative risk measures**

    Relative measures describe the proportional difference between groups.

    Relative risk shows whether something works.

    Common examples:
    - Hazard ratio (HR)—time-to-event outcomes.
    - Risk ratio (RR)—cumulative incidence.
    - Odds ratio (OR)—case-control or logistic regression.
    - Relative risk reduction (RRR).

      These measures are useful for:
    - Comparing groups statistically.
    - Meta-analyses.
    - Understanding direction and magnitude of association.
    - But they do not tell you how big the effect is in real terms.
    - Odds ratios can substantially overestimate perceived risk when outcomes are common and should be interpreted with caution.
  - **Absolute risk measures**

    Absolute measures describe the actual difference in outcomes between groups.

    Absolute measures answer the question: How many patients are actually helped or harmed?

    Absolute risk shows how much an effect matters, providing clinical meaning.

    Common examples:

- Absolute risk difference (ARD).
- Event rates (e.g., 5-year survival, toxicity rate).
- Number needed to treat (NNT).
- Number needed to harm (NNH).

– Examples

Example 1: Relative risk alone (incomplete)

- "Treatment A improved overall survival compared with treatment B (HR 0.80, $p = 0.03$)." This sounds impressive but lacks context.
- Improved version (relative + absolute): "Treatment A was associated with improved overall survival compared with treatment B (HR 0.80, 95% CI 0.65–0.98, $p = 0.03$), corresponding to a 5-year survival of 85% vs 80% (absolute difference 5%; NNT = 20)."

Example 2: Odds ratio vs absolute risk

- "The odds of grade ≥3 toxicity were higher with treatment A (OR 2.0, $p = 0.01$)." This may overstate harm.
- Improved version: "Grade ≥3 toxicity occurred in 4% of patients receiving treatment A and 2% receiving treatment B (OR 2.0, 95% CI 1.2–3.3), corresponding to an absolute risk increase of 2% (NNH = 50)."

Sections

- Paragraph 1
  - Total sample size.
  - Eligibility, inclusion, exclusion.
  - Length of study period (e.g., years).
  - Patient characteristics and demographics: age, gender, etc.

    Table 1 and/or Figure 1 present descriptive data about patients.
  - Treatment and exposure information.
  - Details specific to study design:

    Randomized conditions:
    - Describe numbers by condition and refer to the CONSORT or similar diagram.
    - If applicable, describe study response rates.
    - Describe construction of the analytic sample (i.e., numbers excluded from the analysis).

Retrospective cohort study:
- Number of patients.
- Patient characteristics.

Systematic review:
- How many studies included, where they were published, common features of patients.
- Mention the PICOS, PRISMA, MOOSE frameworks.
- Paragraph 2-n

– Discuss results as they relate to aims of the study, sequentially.
– Mention all tables and figures, sequentially.
  "Table 2 lists…"
  "Figure 1 illustrates…"
– Mention key takeaways from the tables/figures.
– If basic science study, start with in vitro, then move to in vivo.
– If clinical study, start with outcomes/efficacy, then move to toxicity.
– Be clear in what was measured among groups.
– If you need more room to describe what you did, but it doesn't fit, refer to it in a supplement.

Common errors
- ***Presenting results in order that is different from aims.***
- ***Not referencing all tables and figures.***
- ***Copying and pasting the figure legend into results.***
- ***Putting in references. Unless you have a systematic review, you don't need references (generally).***
- ***Being too wordy in descriptions and not quantifying the data***
  – ***e.g., "There were 200 patients. The patients were treated from 1990 to 2000. Of the 200 patients included, 100 (50.00%) of the patients were male. The median age of the patients was 50. Interquartile range for the age was 25–75."***
  – ***Could write: "There were 200 patients (years 1990–2000), 50% were male, median age 50 (interquartile range, 25–75)."***
- ***New variables or analyses are mentioned for the first time in this section. Cross check that Abstract, Introduction, Methods, and Results all mention the same key variables in the same order.***
- ***Discussing the results vs other studies.***
- ***Common errors regarding absolute and relative risk***
  – ***Reporting only p-values.***
  – ***Reporting only hazard ratios or odds ratios.***

  - ***Using relative risk to imply clinical importance.***
  - ***Omitting baseline risk.***
  - ***Burying absolute risks in supplements.***

How to handle null results:

Null results are not failures. They are a normal and valuable outcome of medical research. When written clearly, analyzed rigorously, and framed appropriately, studies with null findings are publishable and contribute meaningfully to the scientific literature. However, they are more difficult to publish than results that show a difference.

- Why null results are important:
  - Prevent duplication of ineffective or harmful interventions.
  - Refine clinical decision-making.
  - Inform future trial design and power calculations.
  - Reduce publication bias and exaggerated effect estimates.
- Null results are often due to:
  - Insufficient statistical power.
  - Small effect sizes.
  - Heterogeneous patient populations.
  - Measurement limitations.
  - True absence of a clinically meaningful effect.
- Null studies are more likely to be published when:
  - The research question is clinically important.
  - The study design is rigorous.
  - Endpoints were prespecified.
  - Data quality is high.
  - The analysis is transparent.
- Common mistakes with null studies
  - Abandoning the project prematurely.
  - "Data dredging" to find a positive result.
  - Overemphasizing post-hoc subgroup analyses.
  - Using emotionally loaded language.
  - Hiding null results in supplements.
- In the discussion:
  - State clearly that the primary outcome was null.
  - Explain plausible reasons for the finding.
  - Compare results with prior studies without defensive language.
  - Address power and limitations honestly.

  - Discuss clinical relevance, not just statistical significance.
  - Do not conclude equivalence unless the study was explicitly designed and powered as an equivalence or noninferiority study.

Making Tables

When to create:

- The tables are the first things you generate, along with the figures.
- **Note**: this is one of the first parts of the paper that reviewers read. If this part is not clear, they will reject your paper. The tables are not technically part of the results section (they are usually at the end of the word doc), but I put this section here because the tables are commonly referenced in the results.

Goal of this section:

- To present data coherently.

How to create:

- Pick ~3–6 tables and figures TOTAL for your paper (depending on editorial constraints).
  - If you have other data that is not important enough to make it here, put it in a supplementary file.
- Table 1 is usually patient characteristics.
- Table 2 and 3 are usually results that complement the figures, but not the same thing as the figures in number format.
- Tables and figures tell a story, i.e., they should address the objective laid out in the abstract and last paragraph of introduction.
- Tables should compare groups with respect to characteristics.
- Size: Tables should be $>2 \times 2$ (too small, can be said in text) but $<\sim 10 \times 10$ (or some large number) in cells. Most Tables have at several columns for the groups being compared $\times$ at least three to four rows for the variables in those groups.
  - Subsequently, each table is one to two pages. If your table is <half a page, you probably don't need a table, just write out what you want to say.
- Tables should not have a table in a table, like where the rows or columns suddenly change the data they are showing.
- Margins are minimal size, e.g., 0.01 cm.

- Two to four significant figures are used. Sig figs are consistent.
- Font is ~8–10 size minimum.
  - Journals usually won't let you make it smaller than that.
- Tables are not XLS files.

If there are references in your tables, keep tables part of the main word document, so that your referencing software auto updates them. If in a separate file, they won't be updated.

Common errors:
- ***The reader would not generate the same conclusion as you after reading the abstract, tables, and figures.***
- ***Tables are not related to the hypothesis, purpose, goal of the paper.***
- ***Tables too basic or too complex.***
  - ***Table that is too simple: a single column of random variables of all patients in the study. A different column shows % instead of n.***
  - ***Table that is too complex: multiple subgroups are presented and all variables relevant to those subgroups are presented across several tables.***
- ***Tables not referenced in paper, or are referenced out of order.***
- ***Alternating number of rows or columns ("table under a table").***
- ***Difficulty finding what is statistically significant.***
- ***Inconsistent significant figures.***
- ***Tables don't fit because the margins are too wide.***
- ***Using mean and SD when you should have used median and IQR; mixing up SD vs IQR.***

Making Figures

When to create:
- The figures are the first things you generate, along with the tables.
- **Note**: this is one of the first parts of paper that reviewers read. If this part is not clear, they will reject your paper. The figures are not technically part of the results section (they are usually in a separate PDF), but I put this section here because the figures are commonly referenced in the results. Similarly, the Figure legends are usually at the end of the manuscript in the DOCX file, and not in the PDFs of the figures.

Goal of this section:

- To present data coherently.
- A picture is worth a thousand words, so the figure should be displaying thousands of numbers or themes that could not be explained simply.

How to create:

- General
  - For most projects, save figures in a PPTX file (not embedded in DOCX, not JPG).
    Slide 1 is Figure 1, slide 2 is Figure 2, etc.
    Supplementary figures can have their own PPTX, PRN.
    Titles and legends are separate and should in a DOCX, usually at the end of manuscript.
    Consider Adobe Illustrator, Photoshop, GraphPad Prism PRN.
  - To convert PPTX to another file type: "Save as… PDF"; "Save as… JPG", but remember to modify registry/output resolution to be high (e.g., 300 DPI), so there is no pixelation/grainy image.
  - For most manuscripts, the # of tables + figures should = 1–5 (depending on journal guidelines).
    Each figure should provide overview of one core message or goal of the manuscript.
    Panels in the figure can present different parts of the same theme.
    Each figure should save words from describing it in a table or in manuscript text.
  - Keep file size <~1–5 MB so it can be easily emailed, uploaded, opened, etc.
  - Follow journal guidelines, from website.
  - Number of figure should match where it is cited in the manuscript; total # of figures = # uploaded to journal.
  - Do not include tables in figures or as JPGs. And I apologize in advance if this book commits this error.
  - Minimal (or no) abbreviations. If using abbreviations, define in legend.
  - No minor errors: typos, grammar, syntax, changing fonts, inappropriate significant figures, ditzels.

  - Dimensions ~1 × 1, 4 × 3, 16 × 9, as they appear best in the published work and online.
  - "Sentence case": by convention, only the first word of titles, legends, axis labels, keys, etc is capitalized.
- Titles and legends
  - Titles are in DOCX (usually at end of manuscript), immediately before each legend. Titles, legends are not in PPTX.
  - Each title is brief, describing the overall purpose of the figure.
  - The legend tells the reader succinctly (~1–5 sentences) what the x and y axes are, the message of the figure or panels.
  - Title or legend should not be copied/pasted into or out of the results.
- Image
  - Use vectors, not rasters. If possible, avoid copy/pasting JPGs into the PPTX: most biostatistics programs output a rasterized file; MS Office (e.g., Excel, PowerPoint) almost always can include vector; text is automatically vectorized.

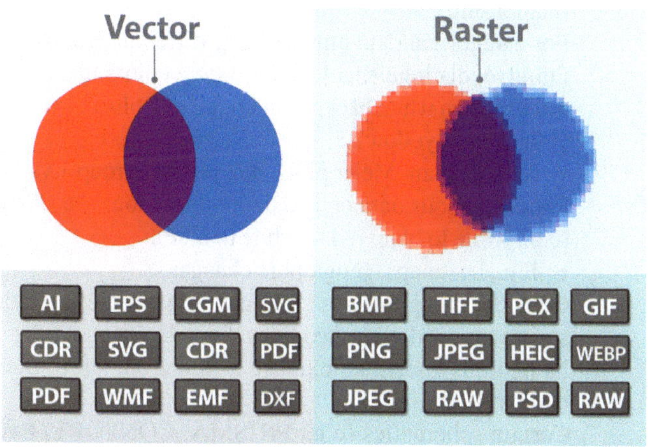

Figure. Vector vs raster

  - Usually: large, bold, black, sans serif font (e.g., Arial).
  - White background.

- Axes:
  Thick, black lines, with labels.
  Independent variable on x axis, dependent variable on y axis.
  Intuitive intervals and sig figs, 10%, 20%, 30%; not 10.00%, 22.5%:
  - Consider log scale if data span 100 + x range.
  - Consider axis break (squiggly line) to show outliers.

  Consider arrows and text boxes to emphasize "better/worse," "favors group A/B" on plot or axis.
- Key:
  Provide if necessary to differentiate groups: e.g., red = group 1, blue = group 2. Make order in key match order of plots.
  Place a portion of the figure that is mostly white space, not showing data. Avoid separating key from plot.
- Colors:
  Color may not be needed if goal is to show simple x–y relationship.
  For categorical data emphasizing different groups: use intuitive, distinguishable, *contrasting* colors that can be discerned on white background (e.g., red, blue, green; not yellow, light yellow).
  - E.g., Kaplan–Meier plots, box plots of group 1 vs 2.

  For continuous data emphasizing transition: use *shades* (e.g., white to blue; red to white to blue).
  - E.g., heatmaps, geographic changes, $.

  Consider using different markers (e.g., circle, triangle, square) or solid vs dashed lines if overlaying plots.
- If the figure is a schematic, make it flow from left to right, then top to bottom.
  Certain schematics (e.g., PRISMA, CONSORT) have downloadable templates.
- If the figure is a representative image, it should be high resolution, emphasizing an archetypal case.

• Avoid
  - Pie charts, as they are too basic for most medical research manuscripts; often, a histogram is better.

- 3D version of a 2D figure, as it does not add information and is difficult to read.
- Figure that could be better summarized in a few sentences or belongs in a table. If the figure is not "worth a 1000 words," it is not necessary.

Checklist for figures:

- Axes are dark/black, in large Arial font
  - If you have multiple plots with the same axes, consider removing the axes labels to avoid repetition.
- Intuitive colors are used: e.g., red for oxygenated blood, blue for deoxygenated blood; pink for breast cancer.
- Panels are used for different parts of one figure (e.g., 1A, 1B).
- Figure legend is not in actual image.
- Appropriate significant figures.
- Minimal (or no) abbreviations.
- Follows journal guidelines.
- Number of figure matches where it is cited in the manuscript (i.e., Figure 1 is first figure in manuscript).
- Number of figures in manuscript = number of figures uploaded.
- No minor errors: typos, grammar, syntax.
- Figures are in a PPTX file.
  - Can save as a PDF or JPG, depending on journal constraints.
  - If saving as JPG, it should be 300 DPI (high resolution).

Common errors:

- ***Figure is not related to the hypothesis, purpose, goal of the paper.***
- ***The reader would not generate the same conclusion as you after reading the abstract, tables, and figures.***
- ***Figure is too basic, e.g., could just be described in text.***
- ***Figure is too complex, too many things going on, should be split into multiple figures or supplements.***
- ***Figure has colors that are not intuitive.***
- ***Figure resolution is poor, or figure contains a low quality JPG that is inserted from another source.***
- ***Data presented in figure when it should have been a table, or vice versa.***

- ***Figure has a title not describing the findings.***
- ***Figure looks like a stock MS PowerPoint plot.***
- ***Issues with typos, grammar, syntax.***
- ***Unreadable font.***
- ***Axes unlabeled or unintelligible.***
- ***Units not appropriate (e.g., reporting follow up as 100, 200, 300 days).***
- ***Figure not cited in manuscript.***

Characteristics of a Good Kaplan–Meier Plot

- Large, bold, black, sans serif font (usually).
- White background.
- Axes:
  - Thick, black lines.
  - Intuitive labels for x- and y-axis: e.g., overall survival, years; not Num_PFS_time.
  - Number at risk on x-axis.
  - Intuitive intervals, e.g.,

    y-axis: 10%, 20%, 30%; not 10.00%, 22.5%.

    x-axis: 1 year, 2 years; not 100 days, 200 days.

    Labeling of the axes matches what is in manuscript text, e.g., "At 5 years, overall survival was 50%."
  - Intuitive range, e.g.,

    y-axis: 0–100, not 90–100.

    - If providing smaller range (e.g., 90–100), consider inset or separate figure.

    x-axis: 0 to all censored data.
  - No gridlines (usually).
- Survival curves:
  - Thick lines.
  - Intuitive, distinguishable, contrasting colors (e.g., red, blue, green; not yellow, light yellow).
  - Consider confidence intervals.
  - Censor marks.

- Interpretation:
  - Appropriate measure and statistical test, e.g., hazard ratio and log-rank test; not rate estimates at a random point estimate where curve separation is maximal or minimal.
  - Clear labeling of tests if multiple curves are being compared.

Making Figure Legends

When to write:

- As you make the figures or when writing the results section.

Goal of this section:

- To describe the key message of the figure to someone who just read your abstract and was wondering if they would draw the same conclusion from the results you presented.

How to write:

- Title of figure should describe the overall message of the figure.
- Present your axes in the legend.
- Figure legend should describe themes in the figure overall and in each individual panel.
- Figure legend should be ~1 paragraph in length.
- Note: Figure legends go into the DOC file. Figure legends should not be in the image, in comments or notes sections of the PPT. Figures themselves should be in PPT or a PDF.

Common errors:

- ***No legend when one would be needed to describe the figure.***
- ***Figure legend is not descriptive, or goes into too much detail.***
- ***Figure legend is in the PPT/JPG.***
- ***Spelling, grammar, syntax errors.***

Using Powerpoint

- Figures made in Powerpoint can be saved as PDFs (a vector file) or as rasters.
- To create an image, copy and paste information directly into a pptx slide and save as a vector ± rasters.
  - File >> save as PDF.
- Change default DPI to >300.
  - To see what your default DPI is, right click your saved file, and check properties.
  - To change default DPI, you must change the registry. Google "how to change increase your Powerpoint to 300 DPI." Change export resolution setting.

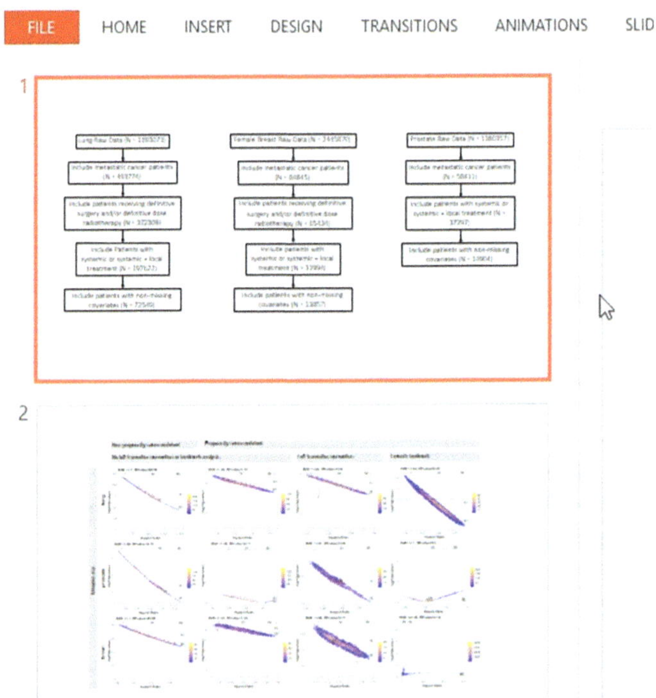

Figure. Powerpoint with each slide as a figure

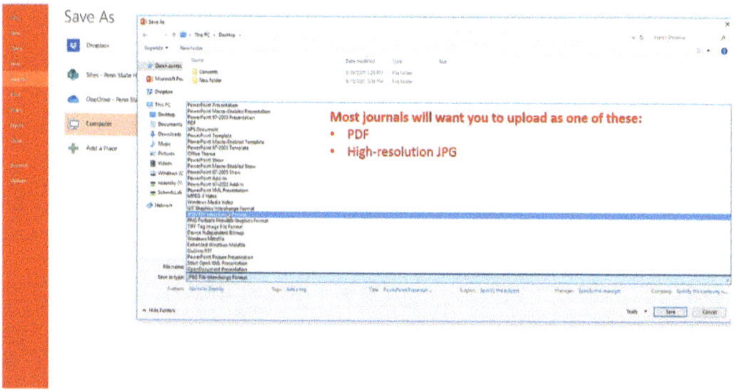

Figure. How to save as a JPG or PDF from powerpoint

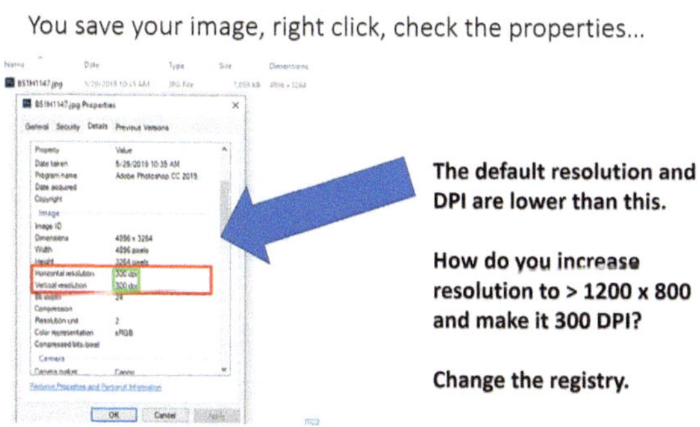

Figure. How to view the DPI of an image

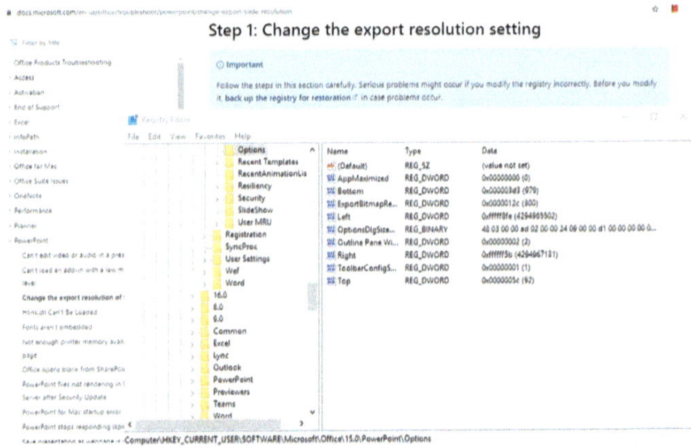

Figure. How to change your registry to change the DPI

Writing the Introduction

10

When to write:

- After results, methods.
- You should already have a general idea of what will be in here based on your prospectus/meeting with your mentor.

Goal of this section:

- To provide some background knowledge, get readers excited in your work, list the purpose of your study.

How to write:

- One double spaced page.
- Stick to two to four paragraphs total aim for 3.
- Provide ~three to ten references, scattered throughout some sentences (i.e., don't have ten references for one sentence). Make sure your references are seminal works for this topic.
- Paragraph 1:
  - Typically, this begins with the big picture public health issue and leads to a description of the specific component of the issue that you are addressing.
  - Describe the overarching problem that your research is trying to solve.

    You could say something like "There are X number of cases of cancer in the US per year," but reviewers of your

N. G. Zaorsky, *Writing a Medical Research Manuscript*, https://doi.org/10.1007/978-3-032-20276-5_10

paper probably already know this, so you may want to jump into more detail already, e.g., "For localized prostate cancer, treatment A and B result in similar survival, but quality of life is better with B. However, there are many subtypes of treatment B, and quality of life differences among these are not well characterized."

- Paragraph 2 (maybe 2 and 3):
  - What do we know about the topic? What is the knowledge gap you are filling? Be careful not to provide a laundry list of previous studies without a critical synthesis and making it clear what the gap is.

    Don't compare your results with other existing studies yet. Save this for the discussion.
  - Focus more on your topic: e.g., "There are multiple treatment options for disease X. Benefits of treatment A include XYZ; benefits of treatment B include XYZ."
  - Leave on a cliffhanger of something missing in the literature and why your study needed to be done.
- Final (usually third) paragraph:
  - Why did you do this study? List your primary and secondary aims/purpose. List your hypothesis (if there is one). Write who this paper would be important to/target audience.

    "The goal of the current study is…"

    "We hypothesize that…" (choose one thing).

    "This work would be useful for X doctors in the management of X condition."
  - *Nature* journals also want you to summarize the paper here.

Common errors:

- ***No hypothesis/purpose.***
- ***Not referencing relevant literature.***
- ***Introduction that is too long (e.g., >1 page). No one is reading your paper to read your intro or discussion.*** *Readers are primarily interested in the question, methods, and findings; therefore, introductions should be concise.*
  - ***Solution: move parts to the discussion. If the discussion is full, then you have too much text overall. You could condense or remove.***

- ***Not a novel question (this is a bigger issue, discuss with your mentor/team).***
- ***Inconsistency among the following*: conclusion in abstract, aims you set out at the end of your intro, first paragraph in the discussion, conclusion in body of text.**

11 Writing the Methods

When to write:

- After you write the tables/figures and results.
- Consider copy and paste from your group's other manuscripts, change parts PRN.

Goal of this section:

- The methods describe what was done to answer the question proposed in the intro and discuss how the results were obtained.

How to write:

- Two double spaced pages. Can have extra info in supplementary files.
- Generally, write this in the order of how you assessed your aims.
  - The first part of the methods section should discuss what was done to address the purpose of your study/answer your research question.
  - The final part of the methods section is the biostatistics component and should discuss the statistical tests.
- General structure of the methods section. Consider the following parts as needed:
  - Study design.

N. G. Zaorsky, *Writing a Medical Research Manuscript*,
https://doi.org/10.1007/978-3-032-20276-5_11

    The Equator Network provides guidelines for reporting findings of different types of studies (i.e., STROBE, CONSORT, PRISMA).

  - Ethics approvals.
  - Patients.

    Recruitment methods.

    Time period.

    Location.

    Inclusion/exclusion criteria.

  - Intervention.

    What are the details of the treatment used?

  - Control group.

    Was there a control group?

  - Outcomes.

    What was the primary endpoint?

    In general, the most important measures for patients:

    - Survival.
    - Quality of life, toxicity.

    Description of included variables and data collection.

    How outcomes are measured.

  - Biostatistics: describe methods of analysis, including:

    Data manipulation.

    Descriptive statistics.

    Analytical statistics.

    Software used.

    Establishment of significance values.

- If you have a systematic review, you need:
  - <u>PICOS table</u>

    Patients.

    Intervention.

    Control group (if any).

Outcome.
Study type.
– PRISMA flow diagram.

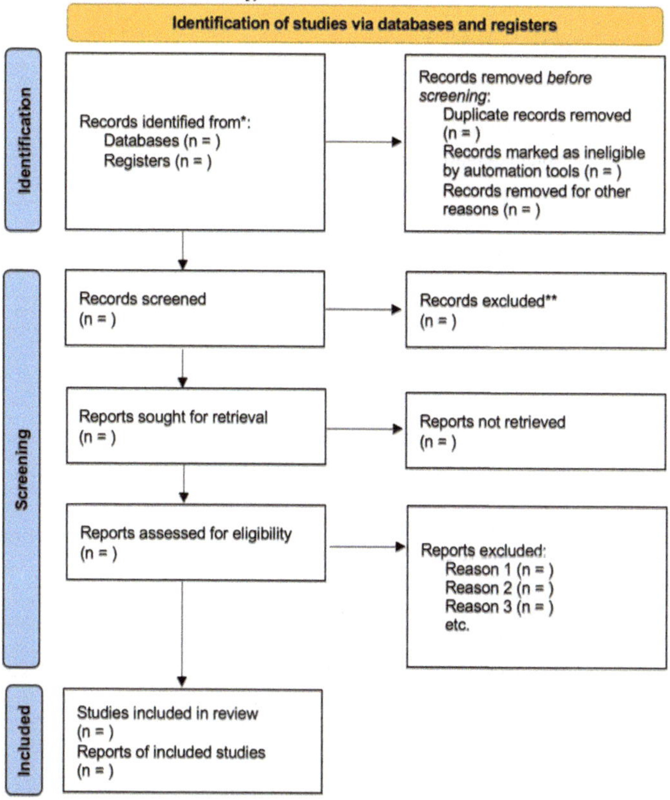

Figure. PRISMA flow diagram. *Consider, if feasible to do so, reporting the number of records identified from each database or register searched (rather than the total number across all databases/registers). **If automation tools were used, indicate how many records were excluded by a human and how many were excluded by automation tools

– MOOSE checklist.

Item no	Recommendation	Reported on page no
Reporting of background should include		
1	Problem definition	
2	Hypothesis statement	
3	Description of study outcome(s)	
4	Type of exposure or intervention used	
5	Type of study designs used	
6	Study population	
Reporting of search strategy should include		
7	Qualifications of searchers (e.g., librarians and investigators)	
8	Search strategy, including time period included in the synthesis and key words	
9	Effort to include all available studies, including contact with authors	
10	Databases and registries searched	
11	Search software used, name and version, including special features used (e.g., explosion)	
12	Use of hand searching (e.g., reference lists of obtained articles)	
13	List of citations located and those excluded, including justification	
14	Methods of addressing articles published in languages other than English	
15	Method of handling abstracts and unpublished studies	
16	Description of any contact with authors	
Reporting of methods should include		
17	Description of relevance or appropriateness of studies assembled for assessing the hypothesis to be tested	
18	Rationale for the selection and coding of data (e.g., sound clinical principles or convenience)	

Item no	Recommendation	Reported on page no
19	Documentation of how data were classified and coded (e.g., multiple raters, blinding, and interrater reliability)	
20	Assessment of confounding (e.g., comparability of cases and controls in studies where appropriate)	
21	Assessment of study quality, including blinding of quality assessors, stratification or regression on possible predictors of study results	
22	Assessment of heterogeneity	
23	Description of statistical methods (e.g., complete description of fixed or random effects models, justification of whether the chosen models account for predictors of study results, dose-response models, or cumulative meta-analysis) in sufficient detail to be replicated	
24	Provision of appropriate tables and graphics	
Reporting of results should include		
25	Graphic summarizing individual study estimates and overall estimate	
26	Table giving descriptive information for each study included	
27	Results of sensitivity testing (e.g., subgroup analysis)	
28	Indication of statistical uncertainty of findings	

Writing the Biostatistics Section

This section outlines how to construct a Methods and Biostatistics section that withstands reviewer scrutiny and supports valid scientific inference.

- **Sample Size, Power, and Study Design Integrity**
  - A high-quality Methods section does more than describe what was done; it demonstrates that the study was designed to

answer the research question in a scientifically defensible way. Reviewers and editors scrutinize this section closely, because weaknesses in design cannot be fixed later in the manuscript.

- **Study Design and Primary Outcome**
  - Begin by explicitly stating the study design (e.g., randomized controlled trial, prospective cohort study, retrospective observational study, case–control study, systematic review) and the setting in which the study was conducted. The design should be clearly aligned with the primary research question and hypothesis.
  - Define the **primary outcome** before describing any secondary or exploratory outcomes. The primary outcome is the anchor of the analysis and determines the validity of statistical inference. Secondary outcomes and subgroup analyses should be labeled as such and interpreted accordingly.
- **Sample Size and Power Considerations**
  - Whenever possible, include a justification for the chosen sample size. For prospective studies, this typically involves a formal power calculation based on:

    the primary outcome,
    the expected effect size,
    the acceptable type I error rate (α), and
    the desired statistical power (1–β).
  - If the study is retrospective or otherwise limited by available data, state this transparently and discuss how the available sample size affects the precision and reliability of the conclusions.
  - Avoid presenting post-hoc "observed power" calculations; instead, emphasize confidence intervals and the magnitude of effect estimates when discussing statistical uncertainty.
- **Data Analysis Plan and Design Integrity**
  - Describe the statistical analysis plan in sufficient detail that a competent researcher could reproduce the analysis. This includes:

    how variables were defined and coded,
    how missing data were handled,
    which statistical tests were used for each type of data, and
    which covariates were included in adjusted models and why.

- Clearly distinguish **pre-specified analyses** from **exploratory analyses**. This distinction is critical for appropriate interpretation of statistical findings.
- When applicable, describe any measures taken to reduce bias, including:
  eligibility criteria,
  matching or adjustment strategies,
  blinding procedures,
  sensitivity analyses, and
  validation of key assumptions.
- Major questions assessed by biostatisticians in the methods section:
  Are the statistics [study design (RCT, observational study), endpoint, etc.] aligned with the research question?
  Can the statistical approach address the question?
  - How is confounding bias accounted for?
  - How is selection bias accounted for?
  - How is missing or censoring data handled?
  - Are there any competing risk events?
- For comparative effectiveness research, discuss methods to balance cohorts and account for bias.
  For prospective studies: randomization (randomized unit, blocking/stratification, allocation ratio, blinding, etc).
  For retrospective studies: propensity score-based approaches (e.g., matching/weighting/stratification/overlap weighting), covariate-balancing weights, g-computation, etc.
- Sample Size/Power analysis (or Precision).
  Trials: primary endpoint, effect size assumptions and justification, variance, α, power, attrition, interim looks/spending functions.
  Observation studies: minimum detectable effect, planned precision (CI width); justify feasibility.
- Specify statistical model, assumptions, and significance level.
  E.g., univariable or multivariable analysis.
  If multivariable, list what variables were included in the model
  If multiple comparisons are being done, is correction (e.g., Bonferroni) used?

Continuous: linear (with robust SEs if heteroskedastic); Binary/count: logistic/Poisson/negative binomial (check dispersion; use robust Poisson for RR); Time-to-event: Cox PH, AFT, flexible parametric, competing risks (cause-specific hazards & Fine–Gray); define time origin, risk sets, time-varying covariates; Longitudinal/repeated: mixed-effects (random intercept/slope) or GEE (working correlation).

Sensitivity analyses. Alternative specifications, trimming/truncating extreme weights, different censoring rules, subgroup analysis.

- Use previously published methods from your group as structural templates, adapting language and details to the current study.

  Consider writing: "The methods have been previously described [reference X]."
- *Nature* journals will ask you to put the methods section at the end, after discussion/conclusion. In my opinion, it's strange.

• **Ethics and Reproducibility**
- State whether institutional review board approval or waiver was obtained, and confirm adherence to ethical standards for research involving human participants.
- Where feasible, briefly indicate how data and code availability support reproducibility and transparency.

Writing the Discussion 12

When to write:

- After you write results section.

Goal of this section:

- To put your study in context of the published literature.
- To compare and contrast your work to published literature.
- To discuss limitations, next steps.

How to write:

- Two double spaced pages, 11–12 point font. Shorter than the results section.
- ~10–20 current, high-impact references; select important historical studies
  - Includes some key references from the introduction.
  - Most paragraphs should have at least one reference.
- ~Four to eight paragraphs
  - 1: Summary of your study in the context of the most important published literature

    Write this paragraph first.

    Summarize the big problem, what has been done to address this problem. Integrate one to two key references from the introduction.

N. G. Zaorsky, *Writing a Medical Research Manuscript*,
https://doi.org/10.1007/978-3-032-20276-5_12

Summarize what your study showed and how it helps to address the problem. Provide one to two memorable numbers or values from your work, highlighting main findings.

- Repetition is good, and you can have the same consistent message throughout the paper.

This is the "hardest hitting paragraph" of the entire paper. You need to summarize results of prior studies, write why your study was important, mention the main findings of your work (with memorable numbers).

Note: this is one of the first parts of the paper that reviewers read. If this part is not clear, they will reject your paper.

– 2-n: Juxtaposing your key findings to the literature

How do your results compare to literature? What are the outliers? What is similar or different? Why might this be the case?

- "we found the most common reason of X was Y, but these authors found…"
- "Prior work has evaluated X, but not Y. We show that Y has…"

Discuss the most important findings in each table/figure, sequentially.

For junior researchers, 99% of everything you want to say, someone else has probably said it better., Paraphrase and cite their work. Find high impact publications on this topic, integrate into discussion, and write how your findings are similar or different vs the literature. Discuss the most important results in the context of literature.

- Use https://scholar.google.com/

Circulate back on themes you brought up in the intro.

- If the primary outcome is null, state this clearly, discuss possible explanations, and explain the clinical implications without overstating subgroup findings.

In some way, the discussion is your editorial/commentary section. primarily read your paper to head about your findings (the results, tables, and figures). The discussion should remain evidence-based and centered on the literature rather than personal opinion.

- Final:
  Limitations of your work.
  - Write this paragraph second.
  - If you could change anything you wanted in the methods, what would it be? Consider: covariates unavailable; selection bias: inclusion criteria, exclusion criteria, sample size; cost; absolute vs relative differences.
    - If retrospective, consider:
      - You don't have certain covariates.
      - There is selection bias.
    - Randomized studies needed.
    - Small sample size.
    - Not representative of the broader population.
    - If meta analysis, you probably don't have individual patient level data.
  - Explain why they aren't fatal flaws, and then end with a positive angle. Be honest, not misleading.
  - Write this after the first paragraph, or first, if you don't know what to put into first paragraph.

  Future directions: can be a separate paragraph or with limitations. What should be done now that your study has been done? Consider ongoing clinical trials.
- Conclusion
  - Sometimes a separate section, sometimes integrated at the end of discussion.
  - Three to five sentences of your core findings, which are similar to the first paragraph of the discussion, and implications of the study.

***Common errors*:**
- ***Inconsistent core message among these parts:***
  - ***Primary aim, hypothesis, goal in the abstract, and last paragraph of the introduction.***
  - ***Results section.***
  - ***First paragraph of discussion.***
  - ***Conclusion.***
- ***Not listing limitations of your work.***
- ***References*:**
  - ***Too few, not putting findings in context.***

  - *Not relating findings to references in introduction.*
  - *Too many references (e.g., >5–10) for a sentence.*
- *Jumping tenses.*
- *Going off into tangents about results.*
- *Too long (e.g., >2 pages, or longer than results section), typically because:*
  - *Presenting or repeating the results verbatim. Instead, find the broad brushstrokes in the findings and compare these findings to published literature. Reference supplements as needed.*
  - *Going in too many tangents about published literature that do not apply to the current study*
  - *Wordy writing, paragraphs >~5 sentences (~half a page).*
- *Misstating or misinterpreting how the current study fits into the larger body of literature within the space.*
- *Not clearly stating how this study adds to the current knowledge gaps/unmet needs.*
- *Overstating results, not appropriately considering the limitations of the current study. No study is perfect, lean into the limitations and discuss how they can be overcome in future studies.*
- *Grammar, syntax, spelling.*

13 Writing the Conclusion

When to write:

- After you write results and discussion sections.

Goal of this section:

- To summarize the core finding(s) of your work.

How to write:

- Write the most salient findings of your work.
- You could probably copy and paste it from the results section.
  - Hint: repetition is good. If reviewers see a consistent message in your paper (i.e., here, in the first paragraph of discussion, in your abstract), they will like it more than seeing inconsistent conclusions/messages.

Common errors:

- ***Inconsistency among the following: conclusion in abstract, aims you set out at the end of your intro, first paragraph in the discussion, conclusion in body of text.***
- ***Presenting known background information.***
- ***Presenting/alluding to things you did not study in your work.***
- ***Esoteric abbreviations.***
- ***Saying "X was higher than Y" (if stating this, just provide the raw number comparison, CI, p value).***

N. G. Zaorsky, *Writing a Medical Research Manuscript*, https://doi.org/10.1007/978-3-032-20276-5_13

- ***Too long, e.g., >3–5 sentences.***
- ***Presenting random findings from your work, not related to the core finding.***

14 Writing the References

When to write:

- The references will be done for you with reference manager software.

Goal of this section:

- To reference literature, allow readers to find the related papers, books, etc.

How to write:

- Your reference page needs to be perfect, i.e., no typos, rogue characters, grammar/syntax errors, font changes, etc.
- Every statement in a manuscript should be supported by the strongest available evidence. References are not decorations; they are the evidence supporting your claims.
- The devil is in the details. If editors/reviewers see issues with your references (easy fixes), they will not trust the quality of your research.
- Choose references carefully. High impact papers often have high impact references (impact not always equal journal IF). Strong manuscripts cite the most relevant and influential references available.
  - To pick references, you should consider citing:
    Guidelines.
    Highly cited articles (look at the google scholar citations).
    Recent articles (in past 10 years).
    Review articles.

N. G. Zaorsky, *Writing a Medical Research Manuscript*,
https://doi.org/10.1007/978-3-032-20276-5_14

Papers, and not book chapters.
Hint: go to google scholar and type in the thing you are writing about.
- Sometimes, one can use an abstract that was presented at a meeting, assuming the publication is pending.
- However, one should almost never use wikipedia, random website, blog, etc.
- Consider referencing clinical trials in progress, registered on clinical trial registry websites, like http://clinicaltrials.gov. You can download the reference and import into EndNote.

- Use EndNote, Zotero, Mendeley, Papers (or another reference manager).
  - See separate section.
- Check the journal website for details on reference limit, formatting.
- Most reference managers will automatically convert formatting from one journal to another.
- For every sentence that has a reference, the reference should support exactly what the sentence is saying.
- Any references presented in tables should also be in the body of the manuscript.
  - For example, you have a table of studies related to yours, and you juxtapose your work to these in the discussion section.
  - If you use ref manager, it will update manuscript and tables all at once.
- References in each section of the manuscript:
  - Self-citation:
    Appropriate when referencing your own prior methods or foundational work. Not appropriate to pad your reference list. Rule of thumb: self-citations should be <20% of your references.
  - Preprints:
    Preprints (e.g., medRxiv) may be cited but label them as such. If since published, cite the published version. Some journals do not accept preprint citations.
  - DOIs:
    Include DOIs whenever available. Many journals now require them. Most reference managers auto-populate DOIs via PubMed; verify before submission.

  - Citation propagation error:
    Do not cite a paper based on how someone else cited it—read the original. If you cite a specific number, verify it against the source.
  - Book chapters:
    Peer-reviewed articles are generally preferred over book chapters, as they are indexed more reliably. Book chapters are acceptable when they are the definitive source on a topic.
  - Intro:
    For primary research manuscript, the intro usually has ~5–10 references.
    The second paragraph of the intro presents the gap in the literature in previous work. You will only need a few references here.
  - Discussion:
    In the discussion section, circle back around to some of the references you presented in the intro.
    What was the gap in the literature? What have your results shown? Are your results in line to what others have presented?
  - Methods:
    Consider referencing stats papers, software, stats website, package, version, etc.
    Biostatistics references are key, especially if your paper depends heavily on the biostats.
  - Most primary research articles do not have references in the results section.
- The results section is meant for data that you obtained.
  - The abstract of the paper should not have references.
  - The conclusion of your manuscript should similarly (in most cases) not have references. The conclusion is meant to summarize what you found.
- Number of references
  - If you are near the reference limit, you might cut some out. Ref managers can tell you # times each is used.
    e.g., EndNote: R click, edit citation, more…
    References used only once may be the easiest to cut.

Common errors:

- *Formatting is poor*
  - *No title, journal name, pages, etc.*
  - *Organization name is interpreted by referencing program as author.*
- *Not quoting relevant literature, e.g.,*
  - *Guidelines.*
  - *Highly cited articles.*
  - *Recent articles.*
  - *Articles, not book chapters (when possible).*
  - *Reference is too low impact/never been cited/in a journal no one has heard about.*
  - *Solution: Search* Google scholar *for topic you are interested in, it will sort relevant references by how many times they're cited.*
- *Wrong references, reference has nothing to do with sentence.*
- *Reference formatting is incorrect, e.g., EndNote sometimes thinks an organization is a person, like the World Health Organization becomes "Organization, W.H."*
- *Reference in manuscript, but not here.*
- *Reference listed here, but not in manuscript.*
- *Referencing too many studies in the intro (e.g., >10–20), and then only a few in discussion.*
- *Referencing too few studies, e.g., <10 for full manuscript.*

15 Writing the Abstract

When to write:

- Last, after you wrote everything else.
- **Note**: this is one of the first parts of the paper that reviewers read. If this part is not clear, they will reject your paper.

Goal of this section:

- To summarize your study. The abstract should succinctly describe the context and purpose of your study, the methods, and the most important results and conclusions.
- The abstract is like a haiku, it squeezes a lot of information into as few words as possible.

General overview:

- ~One double spaced page, generally <250–300 words (depending on journal).
- Copy and paste key lines from your paper, condense as needed (hence, why you write it last).
- Structure the abstract into four parts.
  - Introduction and purpose:

    Brief, pertinent background.

    What is the purpose, question, hypothesis, aim, or objective?

N. G. Zaorsky, *Writing a Medical Research Manuscript*,
https://doi.org/10.1007/978-3-032-20276-5_15

- Methods:
  What was done to address the question?
  How was this done?
- Results:
  This is the most important part of the abstract.
  What were the findings from your methods, in relation to the question?
  Be quantitative (use numbers).
- Conclusion:
  What is the interpretation of the results, in relation to your question?

- The results section is the most important part, so start here. It needs numbers, *p* values. The results section should be super condensed, fitting in as much info as possible.
- If in doubt, length of sections should be: results > methods > intro/conclusion.
- Conclusion can mention something about future work, but don't go overboard/overstate findings.
  - Anything in the conclusion should be in the results.
- Do not use references.
- AI tools may assist with condensation and grammar, but authors should independently verify all numerical results, statistical values, and conclusions.
- Graphical/visual abstracts:
  - Many journals (e.g., Lancet family, Annals of Surgery, Cell) now require or encourage a graphical abstract—a single-panel visual summary of the study's key findings. This is distinct from the "central figure" mentioned above. Check journal requirements early, as these often need to be created in specific dimensions and formats.
- Structured vs. unstructured abstracts:
  - Most clinical journals use structured abstracts (labeled sections), while many basic science and general science journals (Nature, Science, PNAS) use unstructured, single-paragraph abstracts. The journal comparison table below illustrates this distinction.

Background and introduction

- In one to two sentences:
  - Provide a brief, pertinent background, highlighting missing knowledge gap.
  - For most medical meetings, reviewers will already have basic understanding of the field.
  - If tight on characters, cut this section out.
- In one sentence, end with the overarching purpose, hypothesis, aim, or objective
- *Good:*
  - *"The hypothesis is that treatment A improves survival vs treatment B."*
  - *"The purpose of this work is to characterize epidemiology of X cancer."*
  - *"We hypothesize that inhibition of X will lead to increased infiltration of T cells."*
- ***Bad:***
  - ***"We wanted to look for variables that correlate with survival."***
    This is a "fishing expedition."
  - ***"The purpose is to look at survival, epidemiology, quality of life, and prognosis of metastatic cancer patients."***
    This lists too many aims.
  - ***"We did Western blots to look for protein expression after inhibiting protein X."***
    This is too general.

Methods

- The methods section addresses two main questions:
  - What was done to address the purpose?
  - How was this done?
- Methods should be written with the help of an expert in the techniques.
- Major questions assessed by biostatisticians in the methods section.

- Are the statistics (study design, endpoint, etc.) aligned with the research question?
- Can the statistical approach address the question?
  - How is confounding bias accounted for?
  - How is selection bias accounted for?
- The methods section should not:
  - provide spillover from the background.
  - elaborate on everything performed, taking up valuable characters.
  - provide findings/data, which should be in results.
- Use the first part of the methods section to discuss what was done to address the purpose/answer your question.
  - If clinical, consider:
    - Population
      - What were the inclusion and exclusion criteria?
      - How many patients?
    - Interventions—what treatment was used?
    - Control—was there a control group?
    - Outcomes—what was the primary endpoint?
      - In general, the most important measures for patients:
        - survival.
        - quality of life, toxicity.
      - Most other measures are surrogates. If using a surrogate, how is it defined?
    - Setting – prospective, retrospective, randomized, case control?
  - If basic science, consider:
    - Setting - in vitro, in vivo, in silico, etc.
    - Interventions/experiments -
      - Cell lines or tissue/mice used.
      - Drugs or treatments rendered.
      - Describe how you manipulated your model system (i.e., knock-out or overexpress your protein of interest).
      - qPCR, Western blot, flow cytometry, CRISPR, etc.
      - You do NOT need to list all the antibodies/materials you used.
      - Don't forget to mention your controls.
    - # of times each experiment was repeated and the sample size (n).

- Use the final part of the methods section to discuss the statistical tests.

  For comparative effectiveness research, discuss methods to balance cohorts and account for bias:
  - Prospective: randomization.
  - Retrospective: e.g., propensity score matching, stratification*

  Specify statistical model and assumptions.
  - e.g., univariable or multivariable analysis?
  - If multivariable, list what was in the model.

  Specify significance threshold.
  - If multiple comparisons being done, is correction (e.g., Bonferroni) used?

Results

- Results are the most important part of the abstract.
- Succinctly, use numbers and statistical tests to report the findings.
- Consistency in significant figures is important; you will rarely need >3–4 sig figs.
- Depending on the study type and data, consider:
  - For non-normally distributed data (most medical data), list medians and IQRs.
  - For normally distributed data (most basic science data), list means and SDs or SEMs.
- If presenting comparative point estimates, list the 95% CI and/or *p*-value.
  - If low on characters, cut the *p*-values, but not the CIs.
- Use correct estimates in reporting and interpretation:
  - Relative: are HRs, ORs, RRs interpreted on probability scale?
  - Absolute: what is the overall difference?
  - Are differences clinically meaningful?
- Sentences 1–2
  - If clinical:

    Eligibility, inclusion, exclusion.

    Time of study (e.g., years).

    Patient characteristics.

    Treatment information.

- If basic science:
  Controls used.
  Baseline expression of protein or phenomena of interest in your cell lines, animal model, or tissue analyzed.
- Sentences 3–5 address the aims.
  - Some results depend on study type:
    basic science: list experiments in logical order.
    translational: In vitro in vivo in patients.
    clinical: outcomes, toxicities, prognostication, prediction.
  - For all study types:
    Consider descriptive statistics.
    Be quantitative: list specific estimates, CIs, *p*-values, HRs, ORs, RRs.
    Consider using a table to list results.
    Consider study limitations.
    If reporting relative risk difference, report the absolute risk difference as well.
- *Good*
  - *"Treatment A improved survival vs treatment B (HR 0.5, 95 % CI 0.4–0.6, p <0.001), with median survival times of 5 years vs 3 years, respectively."*
  - *"Inhibition of receptor X led to a fivefold increase in gene Y (p <0.001)."*
- ***Bad***
  - ***"There were 100 patients. The median patient age was 65. Half of the patients (50, 50.0000%) were female. The other half were male."***
  - ***Too wordy, inappropriate sig figs.***
  - ***"At 5 years, survival for Group A survival was 50% and for Group B it was 40%."***
  - ***No statistical reporting, just cherry picking a time point. Use HRs and CIs instead.***
  - ***"Results will be presented at the meeting."***

Conclusion:

- The conclusion should:
  - address your purpose, aim, goal, or hypothesis, relating to your results.
  - provide a core take–home message.

- mention potential implications, without overstating findings.
- The conclusion should not:
  - review known information (i.e., what could be in the intro).
  - overstate findings.
  - discuss possible things that could happen with the data.
  - be longer than any other section in the abstract.
- *Good:*
  - *"In patients with condition X, treatment A improved survival vs treatment B."*
  - *"The incidence of X disease is X per 100,000 people."*
  - *[phase I study] "Treatment A may be a viable/safe option, based on toxicity rate of X."*
  - *"HPV E6 binds p53 leading to its degradation in a proteasome dependent manner."*
- ***Bad:***
  - ***"Treatment A is a treatment option."***
    This sounds subjective and does not provide concrete information about outcomes or toxicities.
  - ***"Disease X is deadly and important to study. "***
    This is known information.
  - ***"Gene Z is involved in cell proliferation."***
    This is too general, there is no mention of how, mechanism, or implications.
  - ***Conclusions overstating the findings:***
    "Treatment A improved survival vs treatment B, and treatment C may be even better."
    - ***If work did not assess treatment C, do not mention it.***

    "Treatment A improved survival, and we will next combine treatment A and B together, which should improve survival even more."
    - ***If work did not assess combination A+B, do not mention it.***

    "Treatment A may improve survival, has good quality of life, and is also less expensive than other treatments."
    - ***Listing too many conclusions that were not assessed in this work.***

    "Treatment with X and Drug A led to cell death in vitro. This implies that Treatment X and Drug A may be used to enhance the anti-tumoral immune response."

- ***If you didn't mention the immune response in your results, don't surmise what may happen in completely unrelated experiments.***

Title:

- Titles should:
  - Be relatively short.
  - Integrate the purpose, findings, and/or conclusion.
- Titles should not:
  - Have esoteric abbreviations.
  - Focus solely on methods.
  - State your interpretation of the results.

Journal specific guidelines:

While abstracts generally have a background/purpose, methods, results, and conclusion, some specific journals require a specific format.

- *JAMA* journals have their own style, with ~seven sections.
- *Nature* journals have their own style, with one section (i.e., unstructured abstract).
- Check the journal website to see what other authors did.
- Some have "condensed abstracts" or key points, so adapt this from your main abstract.
- Some ask for a "central figure"—an illustration that summarizes your main findings.
- Some have "highlights", and I would take the main findings.
- Social media message: make it concise about your findings.

***Common errors in abstracts*:**

- ***"I can't meet the character limit."***
  - ***Reasons:***

    Results section too short, but intro and conclusion too long, methods too long.

    Not condensing your sentences enough.

    If you list your CIs, you may not need the p values.
- ***Inconsistency among the following: conclusion in abstract, aims you set out at the end of your intro, first paragraph in the discussion, conclusion in body of text.***

- ***Common errors per abstract section:***
  - ***Background/purpose:***
    Too much background.
    No hypothesis or purpose.
    Hypothesis is not novel.
  - ***Methods:***
    Cannot be used to assess the purpose.
    Insufficient biostatistics.
    Unnecessary details.
  - ***Results:***
    Insufficient quantification of the data, e.g., no estimates, CIs, p-values.
    Out of logical order.
  - ***Conclusion:***
    Does not address the hypothesis or purpose.
    Presents known background.
    Mentions something you did not study.
- ***Common errors throughout the abstract:***
  - ***Grammar, spelling, syntax:***
    Jumping tense.
    Typos.
    Abbreviation inundation: Pick 1–2 max and make sure they are commonly used (e.g., AIDS). Abbreviations should decrease word count significantly.
    Undefined abbreviations.
    Sentences too wordy.
  - ***Significant figure issues.***
  - ***"Missing the forest for the trees": presenting all subgroup estimates, all time points, p-values, CIs, etc., rather than focusing on pertinent estimates.***
  - ***Not enough numbers, no p values, confidence intervals, statistical tests.***
  - ***Starting sentences with the word "this."***
    Subject is unclear.
  - ***"Some…"***
    "…of the [patients/sample]."
    "…improvement in outcomes."

Abstract formats for various journals

	Standard	**Nature**	**JAMA**
Structured?	Yes	No	Yes
Word count limit	Variable. ~3–400	~300	~250
Sections	4:	1:	~7:
	Background/purpose	One to two sentences providing basic intro to field	Importance
	Methods	Two to three sentences more detailed background	Objective
	Results	One sentence of general problem addressed by study	Design, Setting, and Participants
	Conclusion	One sentence summarizing the main result (with the words "here we show" or similar)	Main Outcome and Measure
		One to two sentences to put results in general context	Results
		Two to three sentences to provide broader perspective	Conclusions and Relevance
Additional	Journals like Lancet may also ask for "Research in Context" section.		May need key points:
			Question
	Some journals may ask for lay person summary.		Findings
			Meaning

Examples listed below

Standard

Background: Despite the growing population of individuals identifying as sexual and gender minorities (SGMs), cancer incidence in this underserved cohort remains largely unexamined.

Methods: We estimated cancer incidence trends in SGMs in successive social generations using age-adjusted incidence rates from the Surveillance, Epidemiology, and End Results program's 8 and 22-registry database. Individuals diagnosed with cancers of the breast, prostate, colorectal, lung, or melanoma were defined by sex and single age. Projected incidence rates were derived from Prophet until 2050, with projections for Millennials extending to 2053, when they reach age 65. SGM identification rates were obtained from the 2023 Gallup poll.

Results: The number of breast cancer and melanoma cases for Millennial SGMs is expected to exceed all the previous generations, matched at age 65. Breast cancer cases in Millennials are predicted to be 1106% (7613 cases) higher than in the Silent Generation, and melanoma cases are projected to be 669% (1408 cases) higher. Colorectal cancer cases in Millennials are also expected to surpass the Silent Generation by 248% (1589 cases) and surpass Generation X by 76% (927 cases) for prostate cancer. Lung cancer is expected to decrease by 77% (965 cases) in Millennials compared to Baby Boomers. By 2050, Millennials will represent 49% (7805 cases) of breast cancer and 47% (1558 cases) of melanoma cases in SGMs.

Conclusion: Millennial SGMs are predicted to be diagnosed with three times the number of cancer cases as Silent Generation SGMs (4.0 vs 1.4 per 100,000 at age 65), highlighting the importance of targeted screening and prevention strategies.

Nature

Despite the growing population of individuals identifying as sexual and gender minorities (SGMs), cancer incidence in this underserved cohort remains largely unexamined. We estimate cancer incidence trends in SGMs by generation. Individuals diagnosed with breast, prostate, colorectal, lung cancer, or melanoma were included from the Surveillance, Epidemiology, and End Results, 1975–2021. Projected incidence rates were derived from Prophet and SGM identification rates from the 2023 Gallup poll. The number of breast cancer and melanoma cases among Millennials is expected to exceed all previous generations, with increases of 1106% (7613 cases) and 669% (1408 cases), respectively, compared to the Silent Generation, matched at age 65. Colorectal and prostate cancer cases in Millennials are expected to surpass those of the Silent Generation and Generation X, respectively. Cancer incidence among Millennial SGMs is predicted to be three times that of Silent Generation SGMs (4.0 vs 1.4 per 100,000 at age 65).

JAMA

Importance: Despite the growing population of individuals identifying as sexual and gender minorities (SGMs), cancer incidence in this underserved cohort remains largely unexamined.

Objective: To estimate cancer incidence trends in SGMs in successive social generations.

Design, Setting, and Participants: In this cross-sectional study, age-adjusted invasive cancer incidence rates per 100,000 people from 1975 to 2021 were obtained from the Surveillance, Epidemiology, and End Results (SEER) program's 8 and 22-registry database. Individuals diagnosed with breast, prostate, lung, colorectal, or melanoma cancer were defined by sex and single age. SGM identification rates were obtained from the 2023 Gallup poll.

Main Outcome and Measure: Primary outcomes were estimated age-adjusted incidence rates for SGMs by social generation. The projected incidence rates were calculated using the Prophet time series algorithm.

Results: The projected number of cancer cases for 65-year-old Millennial SGMs is expected to exceed all the previous generations for breast cancer and melanoma. Breast cancer cases in Millennials are predicted to be 1106% (7613) higher than in the Silent Generation, and melanoma cases 669% (1408) higher. Colorectal and prostate cancers in Millennials are also expected to surpass the Silent Generation, with increases of 248% (1589) and 34% (546), respectively. In contrast, colorectal cancer cases are predicted to drop 8% (194) from Generation X, and prostate cancer by 49% (2097) from Baby Boomers. Lung cancer is expected to decrease by 33% (418) in Generation X and 77% (965) in Millennials compared to Baby Boomers. By 2050, Millennials will represent 49% (7805) of breast cancer and 47% (1558) of melanoma cases in the SGM population. Prostate and lung cancer will peak in Baby Boomers but decline in future generations. Generation X is expected to lead colorectal cancer cases by 2050.

Conclusions and Relevance: In this cross-sectional study, Millennial SGMs are predicted to be diagnosed with three times the number of cancer cases as Silent Generation SGMs, matched at age 65. Breast cancer and melanoma are predicted to rise in each successive generation with a marked decline in lung cancer. These data may be useful for the development of targeted screening and prevention strategies.

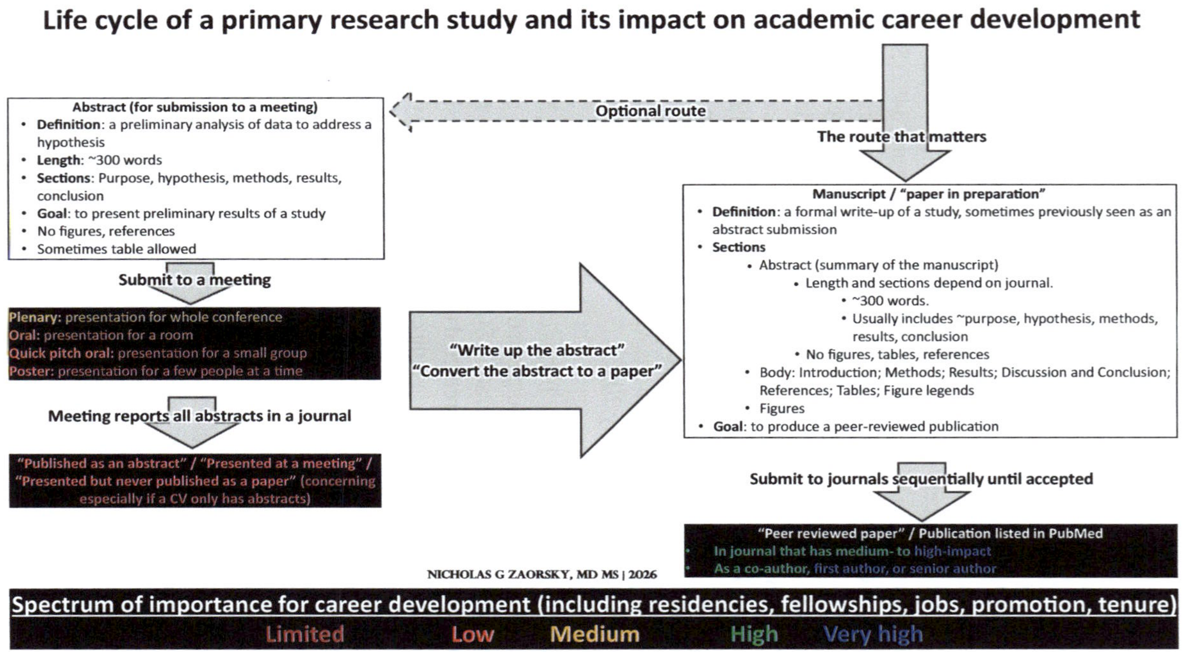
Life cycle of a primary research study and its impact on academic career development
Optional route
The route that matters
Abstract (for submission to a meeting)
• Definition: a preliminary analysis of data to address a hypothesis
• Length: ~300 words
• Sections: Purpose, hypothesis, methods, results, conclusion
• Goal: to present preliminary results of a study
• No figures, references
• Sometimes table allowed
Submit to a meeting
Plenary: presentation for whole conference
Oral: presentation for a room
Quick pitch oral: presentation for a small group
Poster: presentation for a few people at a time
Meeting reports all abstracts in a journal
"Published as an abstract" / "Presented at a meeting" / "Presented but never published as a paper" (concerning especially if a CV only has abstracts)
"Write up the abstract"
"Convert the abstract to a paper"
Manuscript / "paper in preparation"
• Definition: a formal write-up of a study, sometimes previously seen as an abstract submission
• Sections
• Abstract (summary of the manuscript)
• Length and sections depend on journal.
• ~300 words.
• Usually includes ~purpose, hypothesis, methods, results, conclusion
• No figures, tables, references
• Body: Introduction; Methods; Results; Discussion and Conclusion; References; Tables; Figure legends
• Figures
• Goal: to produce a peer-reviewed publication
Submit to journals sequentially until accepted
"Peer reviewed paper" / Publication listed in PubMed
• In journal that has medium- to high-impact
• As a co-author, first author, or senior author
NICHOLAS G ZAORSKY, MD MS | 2026
Spectrum of importance for career development (including residencies, fellowships, jobs, promotion, tenure)
Limited Low Medium High Very high

16 Writing the Title

When to write:

- A working title should be made when you put together the prospectus for your study.
- This working title can be adjusted/refined after the rest of the paper has been written, and according to journal requirements.

Goal of this section:

- To introduce readers to the purpose and/or main findings of your paper.

How to write:

- The title of your paper is the first impression that readers will have of your work. It should include keywords that can be used to identify your topic and search for your paper in databases such as PubMed.
- Some journal articles prefer specific styles of title (i.e., informative or descriptive).
  - Informative titles describe the outcome of the study.
  - Descriptive tiles describe the subject and study design.
- Title words are heavily weighted in PubMed search algorithms, so including key clinical terms (disease, intervention, outcome) directly affects discoverability.
- Many high-impact papers use a colon to separate the topic from the study design or finding (e.g., "Topic: A Randomized Controlled Trial"). This is a widely accepted convention.
- For named trials, include the trial name in the title (e.g., "KEYNOTE-189")—it aids recognition and searchability.

N. G. Zaorsky, *Writing a Medical Research Manuscript*,
https://doi.org/10.1007/978-3-032-20276-5_16

- Good/bad title examples:
  - Good (informative): "Pembrolizumab plus Chemotherapy Improves Overall Survival in Metastatic NSCLC: A Phase III Randomized Trial".
  - Good (descriptive): "Overall Survival with Pembrolizumab plus Chemotherapy in Metastatic NSCLC: The KEYNOTE-189 Trial".
  - Bad (too vague): "A Study of Immunotherapy in Lung Cancer".
  - Bad (too long): "A Retrospective, Multi-Institutional Analysis of the Impact of Pembrolizumab Combined with Carboplatin and Pemetrexed on Overall Survival, Progression-Free Survival, and Toxicity in Patients with Previously Untreated Stage IV Non-Small Cell Lung Cancer".
- Common errors:
  - Esoteric abbreviations that readers outside the subspecialty will not recognize.
- Titles that focus on methods rather than findings (e.g., "A Retrospective Database Analysis of…").
- Titles that state conclusions as fact from observational data (e.g., "Drug X Prevents Disease Y" from a retrospective cohort).
- Too long—aim for ~10–15 words; most journals cap at ~20–25 words.
- Papers with shorter titles get more citations.

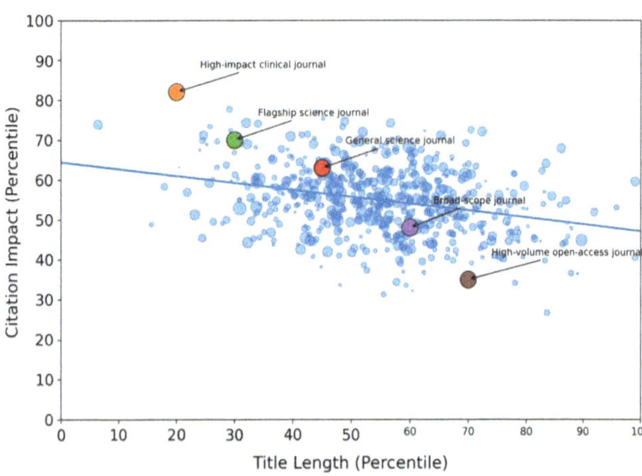

Figure. Citations vs. title length

17 Writing the Cover Letter

When to write:

- As you submit your manuscript to journal.
- The cover letter is a separate file from the manuscript.

Goal of this section:

- To tell the journal editors why this article belongs in this specific journal.

How to write:

- Typical format
  - Paragraph 1
    - Manuscript title
    - Article type
  - Paragraph 2
    - Main finding
    - Why readers will care
    - What is the manuscript about?
    - Why is it novel?
    - Why is it important?
    - Why is it a good fit for this journal?
  - Paragraph 3
    - Required disclosures

N. G. Zaorsky, *Writing a Medical Research Manuscript*, https://doi.org/10.1007/978-3-032-20276-5_17

- "Dear {chief editor's name}"
  - *Note: in Europe, you should say "Professor Doctor…"; in USA, some people just say Dr or Professor, there is not much distinction.*
- Mention the journal name in the first paragraph.
- Why do you think it would be a good fit for this journal? You can reference:
  - Journal goals from their website.
  - Prior publications they have had in this area, and how this builds on those publications.
  - If they are encouraging these types of articles.
  - You discussed it with one of their editors, and they encouraged you to submit.
- In the last paragraphs:
  - Blanket statement I list: *This manuscript has not been published elsewhere and is not under consideration by another journal. There are no previous submissions or reports that may be regarded as redundant publication of this work. All authors have approved the manuscript and agree with its submission to this journal. We are not using any copyrighted information, patient photographs, identifiers, or other protected health information in this paper. No text, text boxes, figures, or tables in this article have been previously published or owned by another party. We have no conflicts of interests.*
  - Suggest reviewers, with location and email address.
  - If you previously submitted it and got reviews back, but ultimately had it rejected, consider including the prior reviews, and point-by-point response letter of how you addressed them.
- How to choose suggested reviewers:
  - Suggest three to five reviewers who have published in the field but are not direct collaborators or co-authors. Use institutional email addresses (not Gmail/Yahoo), as editors verify reviewer legitimacy. Avoid suggesting reviewers at the same institution as any co-author.
  - Requesting reviewer exclusions: Most journals allow authors to request that specific individuals not review the manuscript (e.g., direct competitors, known conflicts).

– Keep this list short (one to two names) and do not provide a reason unless asked.
– Cover letter length: Keep it to one page. Editors review dozens of submissions; a concise, well-structured letter is more effective than a lengthy one. Do not restate the abstract — summarize the key finding and its significance in two to three sentences.

Common errors:

- ***Writing the wrong editor's name or journal name. This is the fastest way to rejection.***
- ***Not suggesting potential reviewers.***
- ***Copying and pasting abstract.***
- ***Forgetting to update the cover letter when resubmitting to a different journal after rejection—leaving the previous journal's name or editor is an immediate red flag.***
- ***Overstating the significance of the work (e.g., "This groundbreaking study will transform clinical practice…"). Let the data speak; editors are skeptical of hyperbole.***

Circulating the Manuscript

18

When you write manuscripts, done is better than perfect. The default deadline to send the research paper to your mentor (assuming you have all data) is 1–2 weeks.

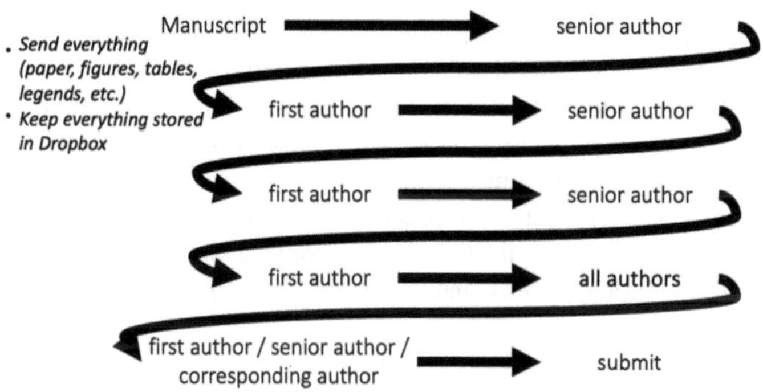

Figure. Circulating the manuscript. The majority of the work is done by the first and senior authors for most manuscripts. The remaining authors are consultants and provide key parts for specific subsections of the work

When you and your mentor are happy with the manuscript, circulate it to the group. If the group is very large, consider using BCC.

- Set a clear deadline. Coauthors should generally be given 1–2 weeks to review the manuscript and provide comments.

N. G. Zaorsky, *Writing a Medical Research Manuscript*,
https://doi.org/10.1007/978-3-032-20276-5_18

- Include the planned submission date in the email.
- Maintain version control. Keep a single master version of themanuscript.
- Avoid having multiple authors edit separate files simultaneously.
- Store manuscripts, figures, tables,legends, and supplemental files in a shared location (e.g., Dropbox, OneDrive, Google Drive).
- Track revisions. Usetrack changes, comments, or version numbering to document edits.
- Save major revisions as separate versions incase prior text needs to be restored.
- Confirm authorship before submission. Verify author order, affiliations, fundingsources, disclosures, and corresponding author information.
- Ensure all authors have reviewed the final version andapprove submission.
- Be prepared to move forward. Some coauthors may not respond despite reminders.
- If reasonable attempts have been made to obtain feedback, manuscript submission should not be indefinitely delayed.
- Keep all files together. Send the manuscript, figures, tables, supplemental materials, cover letter, and any required disclosure forms at the same time.
- Missing filcs crcatc unnecessary delays and confusion.
- Document communication. Keep records of manuscript circulation, author approvals, and major decisions regarding authorship orcontent.
- These records may be helpful if questions arise later.

Sample Email to Circulate a Manuscript

Hello team,

We have prepared the manuscript entitled "XXX" and attached the manuscript, figures, tables, and supplemental materials for your review.

Please review the manuscript and provide any comments, suggested revisions, or concerns by [date]. We are planning to submit the manuscript to [journal name] on [date].

Please also let us know:

Whether you approve being listed as a coauthor.

Whether your affiliation is listed correctly.

Whether you have any conflicts of interest to disclose.

Whether you have suggestions for potential peer reviewers.

Whether you have any additional comments or revisions.

Please review all attached files carefully, including figures, tables, and supplementary materials.

After submission, the journal may contact you directly to confirm authorship or disclosures. Please monitor your email, including your spam folder.

Thank you for your time and contributions to this work.

Best regards,

[Corresponding Author]

19 General Writing Tips

Keys to an efficient writing process

Success is going from failure to failure without losing enthusiasm.

Your writing environment matters. Find where you are productive and capitalize on that time.

Spend as little time writing as you can. Use the tips/tricks for MS Word and other programs to get the job done quickly.

Consider making an outline first. Use short words or phrases to establish the topic and structure of each section, then fill in later. This process will help you build a natural flow that directs readers.

To facilitate productive writing time:
- Choose a time where few people will disturb you, e.g., Saturday at 7 a.m.
- Find a quiet space.
- Avoid distractions such as Facebook, TV, etc.
- Use a dual monitor.
- Use a computer with programs that will help facilitate the writing process. (See chapter on tips/tricks for MS Word and other programs for more details).

N. G. Zaorsky, *Writing a Medical Research Manuscript*,
https://doi.org/10.1007/978-3-032-20276-5_19

If you want to go fast, go alone. If you want to go far, go together.

- Ask your colleagues for help and advice.
- If they can contribute, invite them as coauthors.
- If they talk you out of doing the project for valid concerns, thank them.

The longer a project takes, the longer it will take. Get your work done ASAP. Do not sit on the data.

Set goals and deadlines for yourself. Create structure around the time you spend on your project and stick to them.

I have spent more time not publishing a manuscript than publishing a manuscript.

- Some projects just go fast: get data, write it up, submit it, publish it.
- You don't want projects where you have to go back to the database, pull more data, reanalyze, rewrite, etc.

Ninety nine percent of everything I want to say, someone else has said better, so I use their words.

- When writing the intro and discussion sections, I'm paraphrasing other brilliant authors from other publications, and citing those works directly.

Publishing a manuscript is like doing a history and physical for a patient: your first attempt will be poor, but after some practice, you will be able to do it effectively and efficiently.

Syntax, Style, and Language

e.g. ≠ i.e.

- i.e. = "that is" or "in other words"
- e.g. = "for example"

This/that/these

- Do not start your sentence with the word "this" or "these." Your reader will not know exactly what "this" is and what you are referring to. Instead write out the full noun or subject.

- ❌ "This is the reason we wanted to evaluate drug X for condition Y."
- ✅ "A small phase I study showed improved survival for patients taking drug X for condition Y, and we ran a phase II study to further evaluate its efficacy."

Needless words and phrases:

- "The fact that,"
- "It has been shown that,"
- "Clearly,"
- "Importantly,"
- Starting sentences with "This…"
  - "This is the reason that…."
  - "This makes it difficult to…"

Paragraphs

- Each paragraph should:
  - Be three to six sentences.
  - Be less than ½ of a double spaced page.
  - Have one common theme, introduced in sentence #1.
  - End in one clincher sentence and/or transition to the next theme.
  - Stay in the same tense.
  - Have references as needed.

Abbreviations

- If you use abbreviations in a medical research manuscript, they should:
  - Be common and understood by those outside your field (e.g., AIDS).
  - Decrease word count.
  - Be defined in the manuscript body, and again in tables and as needed.
  - Be used sparingly (e.g., less than 5 in total).

How to condense text and make it provide more information

Initial version:

Many men are diagnosed with prostate cancer. Prostate cancer is deadly. Some men do not die of prostate cancer, but they die of competing causes. Prostate cancer patients can also die of heart disease. Smith et al.[1] showed that patients were at an increased risk to die of heart disease. Prostate cancer patients can also die of stroke. Jones et al.[2] showed that prostate cancer patients have an increased risk to die of stroke. The number of patients who die of stroke are not as many as those who die of heart disease. Nonetheless, the risk of dying from stroke is still high. *Since prostate cancer patients can die of competing causes, it is essential to create programs in cardio-oncology that may mitigate the risk of death from these competing causes. Penn State University has created a program in cardio-oncology.[3] The goal of this program is to minimize risk of death from heart disease and stroke. Additionally, the University of Pittsburgh has created a program to minimize risk of death.[4]* **These programs have been successful in their goals of mitigating risk of competing risk of death. A meta-analysis by Jones et al. recently published showed that these programs decrease the risk by 50%. The effect was highly significant**.[5]

Revised version

About 80% of the 100,000 men diagnosed with prostate cancer in the US will die of competing causes, including heart disease (RR 2.0, 95% CI 1.0–3.0, $p<0.0001$; 30% of competing deaths)[1] and stroke (RR after diagnosis of 4.0, 95% CI 3.0–4.0, $p<0.0001$; 10% of competing deaths).[2] *Two national cardio-oncology programs exist,[3,4] and they mitigate risk of competing causes of death by* **50% (pooled HR 0.5, 95% CI 0.4–0.6, $p<0.0001$)**.[5]

The revised version is specific, providing detailed estimates, including absolute and relative values. It removes unnecessary words. It combines related sentences. It quantifies the data.

File names

- Create a folder with your files. The manuscript file should be called something like {Brief title description} {MANUSCRIPT} {DATE} {Initials of people who edited so far}. For example:
  - "Cancer epidemiology MANUSCRIPT 2025.07.15 NGZ2 MK2.docx"
  - "Cancer epidemiology FIGURES 2025.07.15 NGZ1.pptx"
  - "Cancer epidemiology SUPPLEMENTS 2025.07.15.docx"
  - "Cancer epidemiology COVER LETTER 2025.07.15.docx"
- Do not name your files:
  - "Manuscript.docx"
  - "Paper (1).docx"
  - "Paper FINAL.docx"
  - Or similar
  - You will forget which version of the paper it was, who made comments, when comments were made, which version was most recent/final (there will always be another "final" or revised version), you will not be able to search your computer, or cloud folder for this specific project. Also, file names with parenthesis like (1) usually means you had to save, reupload, etc., and imply sloppy work.

Tricks with MS Word

20

Headings

- Go to View » Navigation Panel.
- In left panel, each heading is a section.
- Clicking on any heading will take you to that section immediately.

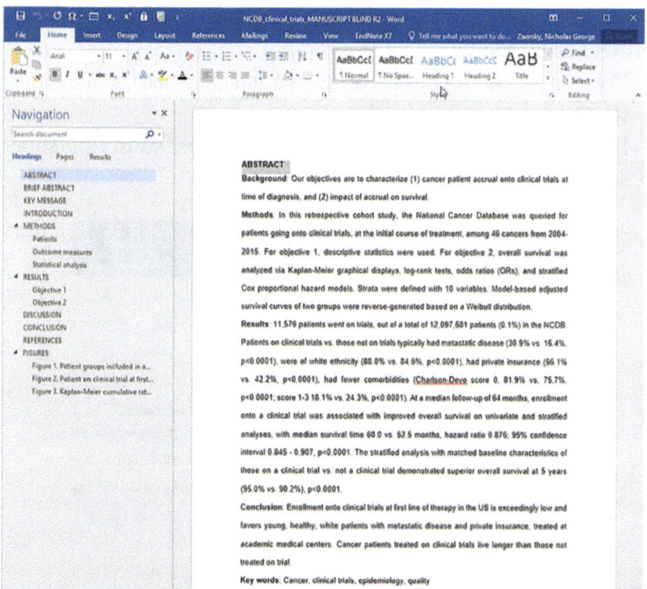

Figure. Using headings in MS Word

N. G. Zaorsky, *Writing a Medical Research Manuscript*,
https://doi.org/10.1007/978-3-032-20276-5_20

Page breaks

- Insert page breaks between sections so it is easier for reviewers to read your paper later.
- Reviewers are humans who are reading your paper after a busy day of clinic. If they can't easily find core components of your manuscript, they will reject it.

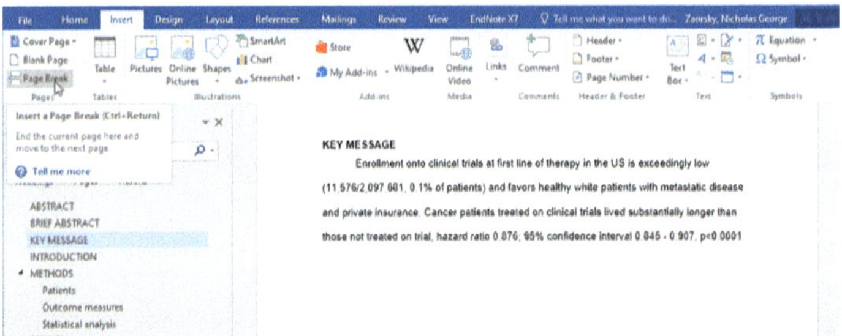

Figure. Using page breaks in MS Word

Quick access toolbar

- You can put all of your favorite commands in here, and then you won't have to search for them.
- I like the symbol button, EndNote functions, subscript/ superscript, etc.

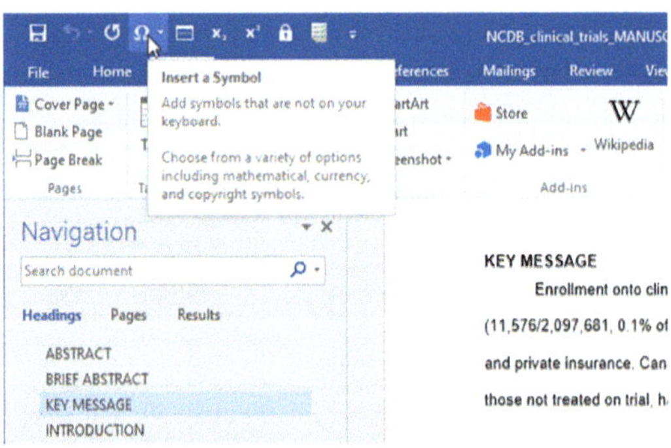

Figure. Inserting symbols in MS Word

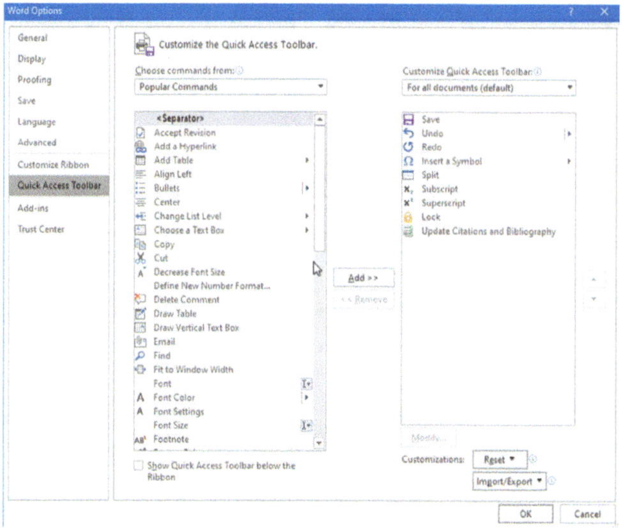

Figure. Changing the quick access toolbar in MS Word

Split window

- Go to View » Split Window.
- Now you have a horizontal divider in your screen. You can read one part of your paper and then check on other parts (e.g., references, tables, figures) while you read the top.

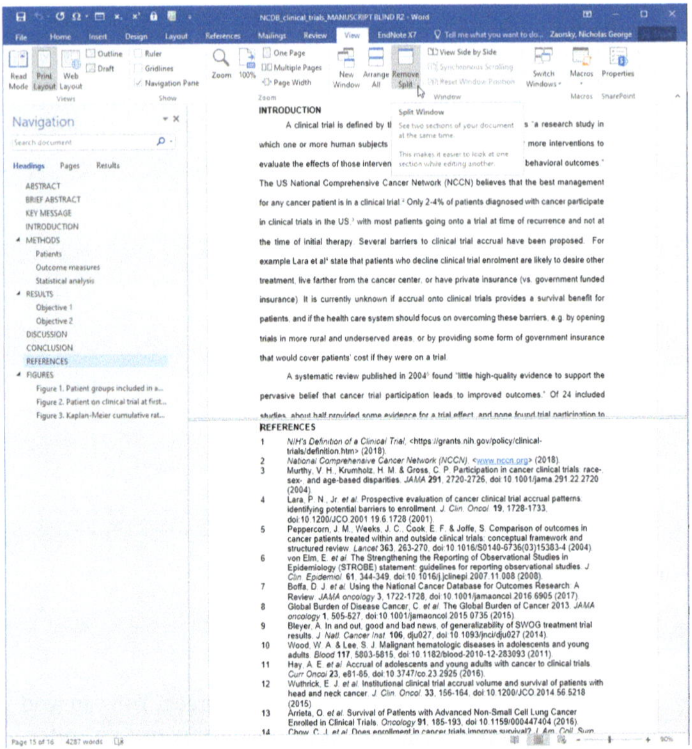

Figure. Using split window in MS Word

Custom dictionary

- Physicians and scientists know 100,000 esoteric words, but MS Word doesn't recognize them.
- Go to Google, type in "medical dictionary in a txt file." Download that file. Add that dictionary to MS Word. No more red squiggles.

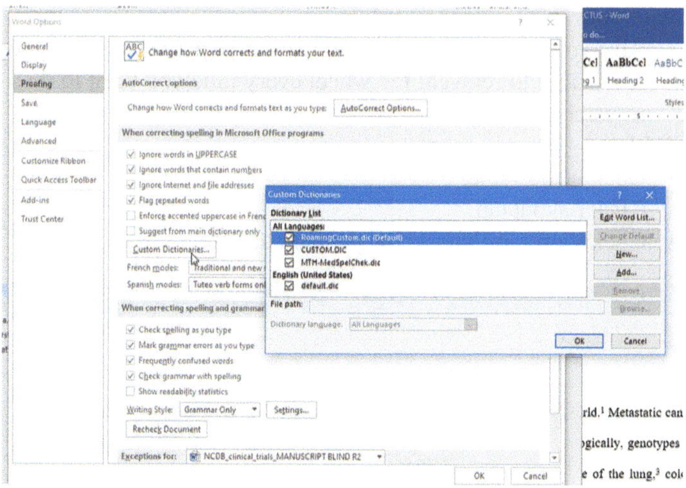

Figure. Changing the custom dictionary in MS Word

Change autorecover save file location

- Tired of losing your files? Save the autorecover location to your Dropbox on all of your computers.
- You can then recover any file from any of your computers.
- Dropbox has an additional feature of keeping temp files for months.

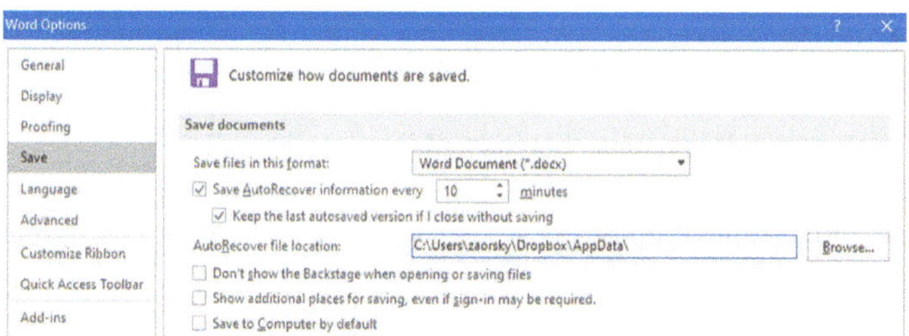

Figure. Changing the autosave location in MS Word

Save your manuscript template

- Save your manuscript as a template for your next work so you don't have to reinvent the wheel every time you want to do a research project.

Tables

- Click in the Table.
- Click Layout tab.
- Click View Gridlines to toggle them on/off.

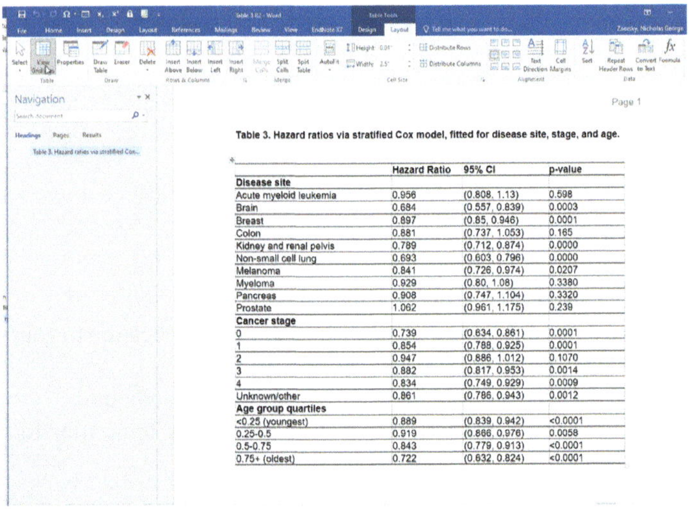

Figure. Changing the table properties in MS Word

- By default in tables, there is padding in each cell.
- Right click the arrow sign.
- Go to Table Properties.
- Go to Options.
- Make the margins 0".
- Now you can squeeze in all of your data.

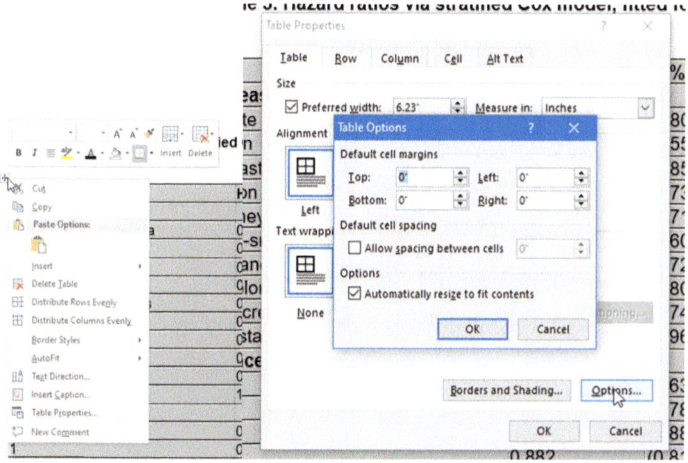

Figure. Changing the cell margins of tables in MS Word

Layout tab

- The Layout tab has a lot of other good features: merging, splitting, inserting, etc.
- You can add these to the Quick Access Toolbar.

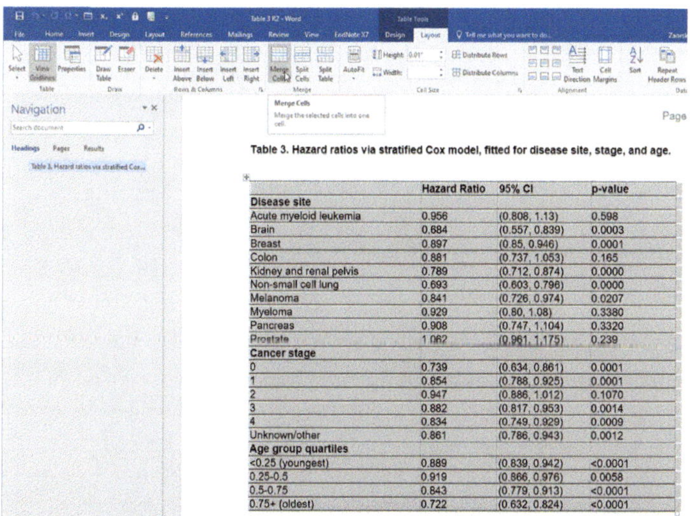

Table 3. Hazard ratios via stratified Cox model, fitted for disease site, stage, and age.

	Hazard Ratio	95% CI	p-value
Disease site			
Acute myeloid leukemia	0.956	(0.808, 1.13)	0.598
Brain	0.684	(0.557, 0.839)	0.0003
Breast	0.897	(0.85, 0.946)	0.0001
Colon	0.881	(0.737, 1.053)	0.165
Kidney and renal pelvis	0.789	(0.712, 0.874)	0.0000
Non-small cell lung	0.693	(0.603, 0.796)	0.0000
Melanoma	0.841	(0.726, 0.974)	0.0207
Myeloma	0.929	(0.80, 1.08)	0.3380
Pancreas	0.908	(0.747, 1.104)	0.3320
Prostate	1.062	(0.961, 1.175)	0.239
Cancer stage			
0	0.739	(0.634, 0.861)	0.0001
1	0.854	(0.788, 0.925)	0.0001
2	0.947	(0.886, 1.012)	0.1070
3	0.882	(0.817, 0.953)	0.0014
4	0.834	(0.749, 0.929)	0.0009
Unknown/other	0.861	(0.786, 0.943)	0.0012
Age group quartiles			
<0.25 (youngest)	0.889	(0.839, 0.942)	<0.0001
0.25-0.5	0.919	(0.866, 0.976)	0.0058
0.5-0.75	0.843	(0.779, 0.913)	<0.0001
0.75+ (oldest)	0.722	(0.632, 0.824)	<0.0001

Figure. Merging cells of tables in MS Word

21 Using Other Programs

How to use EndNote

- Install it and check the MS Word bar.
- Edit\Preferences…
  - Folder locations.
  - Temporary citations.
  - Duplicates\automatically discard duplicates.
- Edit\Output Styles
  - Download your target's PDFs for reference
- Tools\Open Term Lists\Journals Term Lists.
- Save one master library in your Dropbox.
- References:
  - Create references.
  - Import from PubMed
    Search with three names\words; # patients; "unique" words.
- Avoid duplicates.
- Drag references into manuscript.
- Manage your style.
- Click update.
- Managing sequential references.

How to use Zotero

- Go to Zotero.org and press "download" to:

N. G. Zaorsky, *Writing a Medical Research Manuscript*,
https://doi.org/10.1007/978-3-032-20276-5_21

- a) Download the app for your operating system.
- b) Install the Zotero Connector for your browser
  "Install Chrome Connector" → Add to Chrome.
  or "Zotero Connectors for other Browsers" → select your browser → download.

- Pin the Zotero Shortcut to your Extensions bar:
  - Look for the puzzle piece icon on the top right corner of Chrome and press the pin icon next to Zotero Connector.
- Install Zotero.
- Install the Microsoft Word plugin:
  - Open Zotero and press "Install Word plugin" on the popup bar.
- Set up Syncing:
  - To sync your Zotero collections between devices, click "Zotero" on the menu bar → Settings → Sync.
  - Create an account (it's free).
- Create a new collection:
  - Collections are folders that can be used to organize citations for a single project.
  - Click the folder icon on the top left corner of Zotero to create a new collection.
- Add items to your collection:
  - There are many different ways to add items to your collection:
    To add by hand: "New Item" → select the item type → enter information in the panel that pops up to the right of the screen.
    Add by ISBN, DOI, PMID, or other identifiers: select the magic wand button → enter identifier.
    Add by PDF: drag and drop article PDF into your collection, OR "Add Attachment" → "Add file" or "Add link to file."
    Add via Zotero Connector in browser: Pull up the page for your article in your browser → click the Zotero Connector icon → select the Zotero collection you want to sort the paper into → press enter.
    - The PDF of the paper or a link to the paper will show up in "Attachments" under your new entry.
- Add tags to sort and identify your papers:

- Select a paper in your collection → scroll down on panel to right of screen → press "+" to add a new tag.
- If you use Zotero connector, some tags will be automatically created. You can keep these, or remove them by clicking on a tag, then selecting the (-) button to the right.
- You can search by tags in the search bar or filter by tags in the filter bar.

- Add notes to your Zotero library:
  - You can add your own notes about your sources in the Zotero library.
  - To add notes about a specific article, select the article in your collection, and press the "+" next to "Notes" in the panel on the right side
  - You can also add standalone notes to your library. Select the Notes icon on the top bar → "New Standalone Note."
- Using the Zotero plugins for Microsoft Word or Google Docs:
  - To add an in-text citation:
    Click "Zotero" in toolbar → "Add/edit citation" → select your desired citation style → search for your desired paper by title or author's last name → press enter.
  - To add your bibliography/ references:
    Click "Zotero" in toolbar → "Add/edit bibliography."

How to use FoxIt PDF Reader

- FoxIt PDF Reader is a good alternative to Adobe Acrobat. You can convert to and from Word docs, sign PDFs, and search folders of PDFs on your computer for a specific word.
- Highlight.

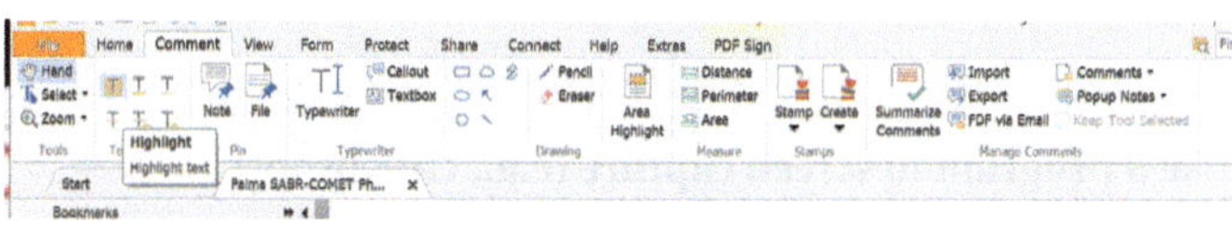

- Insert text, images, shapes:
  - E.g., signatures (as the original JPGs, or drawn on with the program's e-pen).

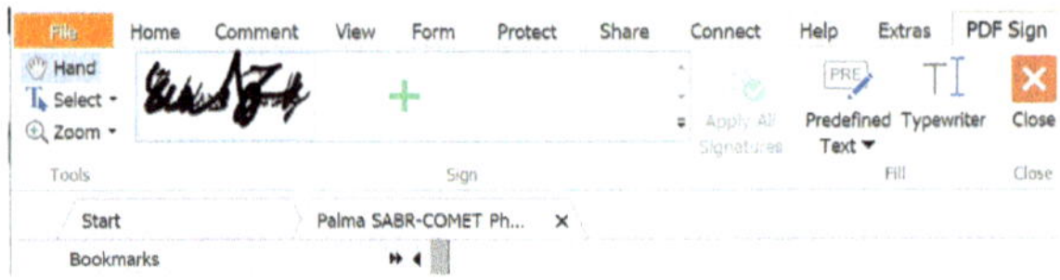

- Search function.

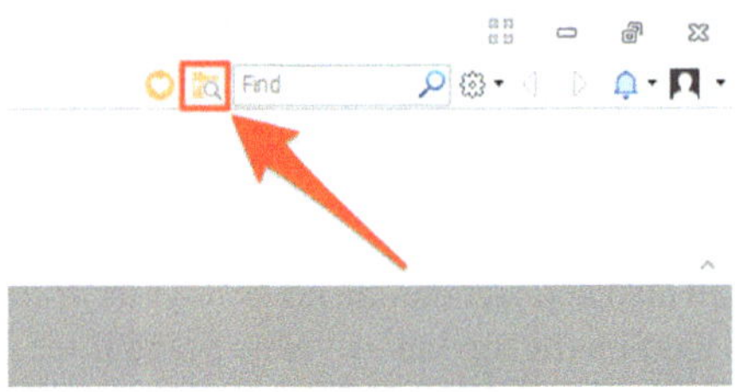

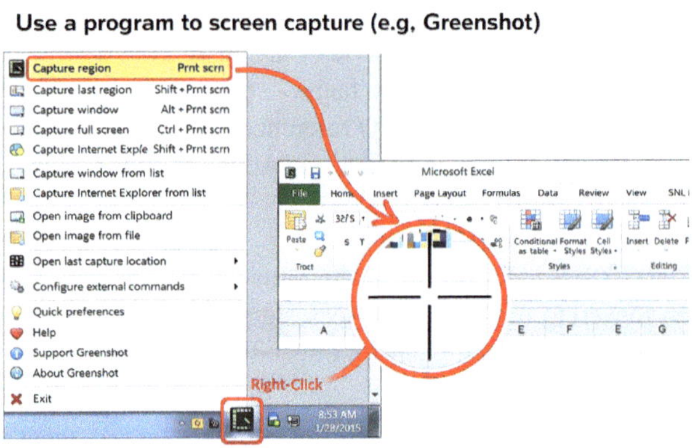

Use a program to screen capture (e.g., Greenshot)

Password Managers

- Password managers like Bitwarden will make it so you don't have to remember your passwords for journals.

22 How to Use Artificial Intelligence (AI) to Improve Your Research Manuscript

Preface

- AI should not be used to replace your writing, but it should be used to make your work more efficient.
- The International Association of Scientific, Technical & Medical Publishers (STM) published a September, 2025 report defining classifications of AI activities. These may be used to determine if your use of AI aligns with journal guidelines.
  1, Refinement, correction, editing, or formatting the manuscript to improve clarity of language.
  2, Writing or drafting manuscript content.
  3, Translation of manuscript text for the purpose of publishing.
  4, Refining or formatting of data reported in the manuscript.
  5, Generation, refinement, correction, editing or formatting of images, diagrams or other figures for illustrative purposes only.
  6, Generation, refinement, correction, editing or formatting of visualizations of research data or results.
  7, Refinement or formatting of code reported in the submitted manuscript.
  8, Assisting with gathering references.
  9, Presentation of any kind of content generated by AI tools as though it were original research data/results from nonmachine sources.

N. G. Zaorsky, *Writing a Medical Research Manuscript*,
https://doi.org/10.1007/978-3-032-20276-5_22

- As of 2025, AI is generally good in two settings:
    1, you know/upload the outcome + prior information; need help with the methodology.
    2, you know/upload the methodology + prior information; need help with the outcome.
- In both cases, you should have prior information, you already know the process and outcome you want relatively well, and you rely on the AI to help with the scut work.
    – **A** is the **prior information**. This could be data, prior papers, prior manuscript from your research group, code, etc.

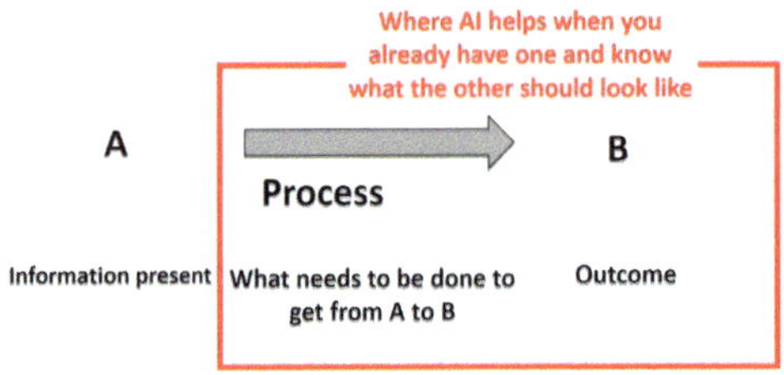

    – **Process** ≠ methods. Rather, it is what needs to be done to get from A to B.
    – **B** is the **outcome**. Outcome ≠ results. This could be figures, parts of a manuscript (intro section; discussion section), COI statements, reference section, criteria for the manuscript (e.g., number of tables and figures; citations for them).

Examples

- You upload **A** and **process**, you need **B**.
    – **Desired outcome**: Generate discussion section.
      Upload: PDFs of prior works cited in introduction, a template (e.g., this book), results section.
      Tell AI: "Evaluate the prior works and our results. Draft a 2 page discussion section where you compare and contrast our paper's results vs. others. Use the template for the section."
    – **Desired outcome**: Create a plot.
      Upload: Your data/results in XLS sheet.
      Tell AI: "Generate bar plots of the data with IQRs. Include IQRs. Perform a nonparametric statistical test (e.g., ordered

chi square, Kruskal–Wallis, etc.), since the data are skewed. Tell me why you chose the test." Note, you should still check with your biostats team, but this can provide prelim evaluation. If using AI for actual methods, then cite in the Methods section.

  - **Desired outcome**: Pre-peer review of manuscript.
    Upload: Your paper. Reviewer checklist from this book (can screenshot). Other related papers.
    Tell AI: "Review this manuscript per reviewer guide book. Tell me major deficiencies in this work, what reviewers may comment on vs. other papers."
- You upload **A** and **B**, you need the **process**.
  - **Desired methodology**: Updated methods section based on prior works.
    Upload: Your prior manuscript and the current manuscript, including results, tables, figures.
    Tell AI: "Generate a methods section like that of our prior paper, but frame it so it would help generate the current tables and figures, based on the goals noted in the intro."
  - **Desired methodology**: Revise formatting from Journal X to Y.
    Upload: Current manuscript after it was rejected from journal X, sample manuscript/instructions from journal Y.
    Tell AI: "We are resubmitting the paper to journal Y, revised paper attached. Make sure we follow journal Y online instructions. Make sure we cite all tables and figures appropriately"
  - **Desired methodology:** Check that calculations were done correctly.
    Upload: A partial version of your results section, methods, code/coding.
    Tell AI: "I did calculations to generate some results, in rows 1–5. Can you double check my calculations (rows 6–100) and equations using the methods and code/coding I provided?"

A Practical Workflow: Using AI to Help Publish Academic Medical Research

NICHOLAS G ZAORSKY, MD MS | 2026

1 **Download my manuscript writing guides from my website or this book**
"How to write an introduction"
"How to write a discussion"
"Checklist before you submit your manuscript"
"How to write a medical research manuscript"
Many others...

2 **Upload your manuscript + guides into AI tools**

3 **Use AI as a structured peer reviewer:**
- Are we following the guides?
- Can you provide peer review before we submit?
- Are there other works we should reference or consider?

4 **Trust but verify.** AI can hallucinate and make errors—it does not replace clinical judgment or mentorship.

5 **Acknowledge.** Disclose AI use. Treat it like statistical software—an assistive tool, not an author.

23 How to Choose a Journal

Choose a journal whose focus aligns with the topic/aims of your paper.

- Most main publishing houses have online tools to help you identify potential journals based on title, abstract, and/or keywords, e.g.:
  - Springer Journal Suggester.
  - https://www.scimagojr.com/

Consider the journal's impact factor.

- Impact factor = [# of citations received in a given year to articles published in the journal in the prior 2 years] / [# of citable articles published in the journal in those same 2 years].
- Excellent: >10–20
  - 10 will be in ~top 3%ile
- Great: ~4–10
  - >6 will be in top ~15%ile
- Good: ~3–5
- Median: ~1
- Unlisted impact factor.
  - New.
  - Case reports/editorials.
  - Recent "open access."
  - Not a real journal.
  - Not on PubMed.

N. G. Zaorsky, *Writing a Medical Research Manuscript*,
https://doi.org/10.1007/978-3-032-20276-5_23

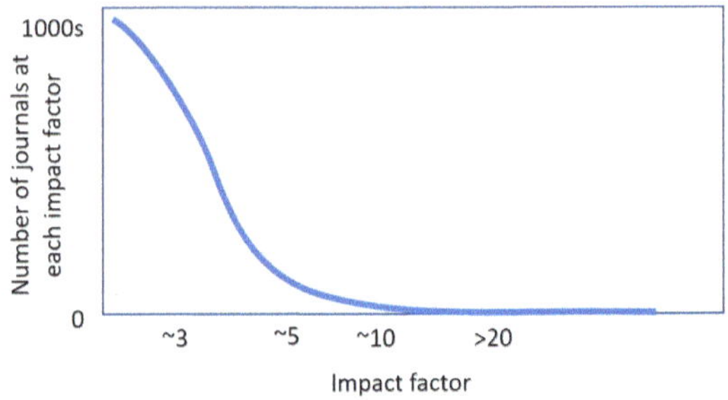

Figure. Number of journals per impact factor

Make a list of three to five journals to submit to, and submit to the one with the highest impact score first. Journal fit is usually more important than impact factor. A manuscript that closely matches a journal's audience is more likely to be reviewed favorably than a manuscript submitted solely based on impact factor.

Only submit to one journal at a time.

For highly specialized projects, authors may contact the editor or editorial office before submission to assess journal fit. Consider reaching out to the editor-in-chief of the journal directly with your DOC and PPT and ask if they would be interested in reviewing this work. If they say yes and it fits with the journal's goals, then submit formally and write that you spoke with the editor. This will save you the time of uploading and then getting instantly rejected.

- If the journal has solicited submissions like yours, write it in your cover letter.
- Writing the manuscript is only 50% done with the research project; it does not yet count on your CV. Publishing A line graph depicting the distribution of journals by impact factor. The x-axis represents the impact factor, with approximate values labeled as ~3, ~5, ~10, and >20. The y-axis shows the number of journals in thousands. The curve starts high on the left, indicating a large number of journals with lower impact factors, and decreases sharply, leveling off as the impact factor increases Alt Text is like applying to college, but you can only submit 1 application at a time. Prepare for rejection. In hockey, one of the basic principles

is to keep the puck on the opponent's side. Similarly, in academic publishing, a manuscript should spend as little time as possible on your desk and as much time as possible under review at a journal.

How to avoid predatory journals

- High tier journals usually do not advertise and rarely will send you invites to submit.
- How to identify a spam research invite (the more of these, the more likely it is spam; 4+ is almost a guarantee):
  - "Greetings of the day."
  - "Dear Dr Prof [Name], [Initial]."
  - "eminent/esteemed/etc."
  - "following up…"
  - "special issue."
  - Invite for review/research/comment/case report/anything.
  - Times New Roman.
  - Random reference to your paper.
  - Highlighting.
  - Colorful font. 2 points if red.
  - Grammar errors.
  - Index Copernicus.
  - Meeting or journal = strange abbreviation.
  - Signed Ms/Mr.
  - Address is random building.
  - You have never heard of this journal.
  - Journal name is similar to a more prominent journal you know.
  - Not on pubmed.
  - Spammy website.
  - Upload website is nonstandard (e.g., not editorialmanager type).

Part III

The Submission and Publication

24 Reasons Why Researchers Should Not Pay Fees to Publish Their Research

1. **Publishing fees are arbitrarily high**. Publishing fees, also termed article processing charges (APCs), are exorbitantly expensive (e.g., $1000s), and they are set by publishing companies. Publishing fees have been rising since the 2000s. Publishing a manuscript actually costs very little (I estimate <$50–100) per article, including creating a website/hosting, and getting the work onto government databases like PubMed.
2. **Researchers are not compensated**. Compensation refers to direct payment (e.g., salary) or indirect payment (e.g., benefits, retirement contributions). The vast majority of clinical researchers are not paid to do their research, since they do it in their limited free time. A small proportion of researchers receive grant funding (usually from government or private companies), and this funding is meant to perform the actual investigation. Researchers may spend hundreds of hours on one research project and thousands of hours on content expertise to do the project.
3. **Editors are not compensated**. Editors of journals, who evaluate the manuscripts and send them for peer review, are almost always not paid. Editors may spend hours handling a paper (i.e., communicating with reviewers and authors) and thousands of hours on their content expertise.

N. G. Zaorsky, *Writing a Medical Research Manuscript*,
https://doi.org/10.1007/978-3-032-20276-5_24

4. **Peer reviewers are not compensated**. Reviewers may spend hours reviewing a paper and communicating with the editors, plus thousands of hours to have content expertise.
5. **Trainees are relatively poor**. Trainees, who are often first authors or coauthors, and the workhorses behind the research, often have to pay tuition while they are doing the research (e.g., medical students pay >$50K/year), live on a modest salary (e.g., residents), and/or they have exorbitant loans (e.g., the median loan of a US medical graduate is ~$220K in 2023), all while working incredibly long hours.
6. **Publishing company revenues are high**. Publishing companies generate incredibly large revenues and have margins larger than most publicly traded companies (e.g., Google, Microsoft). Much of the revenue comes from advertisements and journal subscriptions from libraries/schools.
7. **Researchers have limited rights after publication**. Researchers already sign away their rights to the article when they choose to publish with a journal.
8. **Researchers assume all risks for the content**. After publishing an article in a journal, researchers are still responsible for the integrity of the work, the analyses, etc.
9. **Journals charging to publish are usually junk**. Most journals with publication fees are relatively low quality and/or low impact. Few exceptions exist. Numerous other journals without fees exist to publish a research article.
10. **Most scientific research is noble and thus should not be financially penalized**. Medical research is aimed to improve human quality or quantity of life. If the research being published was in a less altruistic field (e.g., maximizing corporate profit), then making the authors pay may be justified.

25 Finding Reviewers

- It is hard for the editors to find reviewers. The success rate for people agreeing to review is less than 50%.
- You should aim to have ~5 suggested peer reviewers listed in the cover letter and submission website when you submit your manuscript.
- How to find suggested reviewers?
  - Google/PubMed the first and last authors of papers you are referencing.
  - Type in the topic you are researching to Google Scholar. If they have a Google Scholar account, they are probably tech-savvy enough to be interested in reviewing too.
  - Typically, you want younger people, like assistant/associate professors who provide good feedback, especially if you're referencing their papers. Sometimes more senior investigators are too busy.
  - Talk to your mentor and coauthors for their suggestions.
  - How do you find email addresses?

    For unique last name (e.g., mine), you could just put in last name.

    For common last name (e.g., superstar colleague Ming Wang), consider adding institution or coauthor.

    In either case, you need papers where they are first or senior author (usually = corresponding author too).

N. G. Zaorsky, *Writing a Medical Research Manuscript*,
https://doi.org/10.1007/978-3-032-20276-5_25

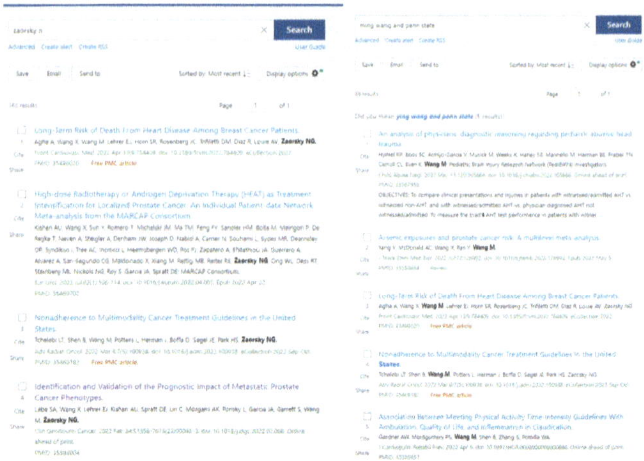

Figure. Finding reviewer email addresses. Click on a publication, click expand affiliations. The email address is usually listed there. If it is an institutional (i.e., .edu, .org) address, then consider double checking Google to make sure this person is still at the institution. What if the email address isn't listed on the PubMed page? You may need to pull up a journal website/PDF

26 Common Errors in a Submitted Manuscript

- Errors in the most important parts of the paper: tables, figures, abstract(the most important parts of the paper).
- Inconsistency among the following: conclusion in abstract, aims you set out at the end of your intro, first paragraph in the discussion, conclusion in body of text.
- Spelling, grammar, syntax errors. These are a surrogate for the quality of your work. If you have any of these in the abstract, there is a high likelihoodreviewers will reject your paper.
  - Using varying terms for the same thing, e.g., radiotherapy vs. radiation therapy vs. RT vs. ionizing radiation.
  - Using varying methods to write statistics, e.g., (95% confidence interval, X to Y) (95% confidence interval: X, Y).
  - No space in between equals sign, commas.
  - Not knowing difference between i.e. and e.g.:

    i.e. = that is

    e.g. = for example
  - Inconsistent significant figures.
  - Spaces, parentheses, brackets where they shouldn't be.
  - Sentences that are too lengthy.
  - Tense jumping around

    CTRL F: am/is/are/was/were/be/being/been.
  - Undefined abbreviations.
  - Abbreviations defined multiple times.

N. G. Zaorsky, *Writing a Medical Research Manuscript*,
https://doi.org/10.1007/978-3-032-20276-5_26

- References outside and inside punctuation (pick one).
- Using too many significant figures, e.g., you have 100 patients, and you write that 66.666% had an event. Just write 67%.
- Idiosyncratic abbreviations or too many abbreviations (e.g., > 3–5 terms abbreviated).
- Paragraphs that are too short (e.g., one to two sentences) or too long (e.g., > half a page). Keep paragraphs to three to five sentences.
- Starting sentences with the word "This/these"

  E.g., "This makes it hard to study prostate cancer"/"this inspired us to…"—the reader will not know what "This" is, and you should just list a clear subject.
- Needless words and phrases

  "The fact that"

  "It has been shown that"

  "Clearly,"

  "Importantly,"

• Not using the "Headings" feature in MS Word, and not using headings/subheadings. Hint: go to "Home" tab, then "Styles", then "Heading 1." In the "view" tab, in the "Navigation pane," the headings and subheadings will appear and make it easier to scroll through your manuscript.
• Not using the "View," "Split screen" function when you write.

27 Checklist for Before You Click "Submit" for Your Research Manuscript

- Cover letter:
  - Lists correct journal, editor-in-chief.
  - Describes why the manuscript is a good fit for the journal.
  - Recommends peer reviewers, including reasons, email addresses.
- Formatting follows journal guidelines from website.
- Objective, hypothesis, purpose, or aim is:
  - Clearly defined.
  - Consistent among:
    - Intro/background of the abstract.
    - Last paragraph of the introduction.
- Conclusion:
  - Addresses the objective, hypothesis, purpose, or aim.
  - Consistent among:
    - Last part of the abstract.
    - First paragraph of the discussion (putting your work in context of what is known).
    - Conclusion in the body of the manuscript.
- Data and results:
  - Quantified (i.e., use numbers, ranges, *p*-values).
  - Consistent among the following:
    - Results section of the abstract.
    - Results section of manuscript body.
  - Significant figures are appropriate and consistent.

N. G. Zaorsky, *Writing a Medical Research Manuscript*,
https://doi.org/10.1007/978-3-032-20276-5_27

- Tables and figures:
  - High quality (no blurry images).
  - Number of each table and figure matches where it is cited in the manuscript.
  - Number of tables and figures listed in the manuscript = number of tables and figures uploaded.
  - Values add up correctly, e.g.:
    PRISMA, CONSORT diagrams.
    Table sums.
- No minor errors, e.g.: typos, grammar/syntax; font; color; abbreviations.
- References:
  - Have no minor errors.
  - Support the sentence they follow in the manuscript.
- Coauthors:
  - Reviewed the manuscript, made comments, approved of submission.
  - Submitted conflict of interest forms.
  - Notified of submission via email.

28 What to Complete on the Manuscript Submission Screen

- Fill out all author names and email addresses.
  - The institutions, departments, phones, etc. don't matter as much.
- Upload the manuscript DOCX file(s), figure files (PPTX or PDF), and supplements.
- Upload the cover letter.
- No, you don't want to publish in color (it costs extra, and color on the internet is free).
- No, you don't want to publish open access.
- No, you don't want to forward it to their open access journal (see Chapter 24), unless it is a journal that can waive the fee.
- Do you want to make it unblinded so reviewers see your name? If available, I usually click yes because I hope reviewers know it's me, and our team does good science.
- Do you want to upload your manuscript to the archive/repository? I haven't done this in the past, but maybe it's fine—you made a breakthrough and want to claim that you did it first. Nature journals offer this option.
- "Build PDF"—will make a PDF of the manuscript files. Send this to your mentorship team (may be all coauthors). This is the file that will be seen by reviewers.

N. G. Zaorsky, *Writing a Medical Research Manuscript*,
https://doi.org/10.1007/978-3-032-20276-5_28

29 Submission Process

Publishing a manuscript takes a long time.

- It is hard to find reviewers (which is why you should suggest some). Holidays, lack of reviewer compensation, mixed reviews requiring additional opinions, and difficulty recruiting all contribute to delays.

N. G. Zaorsky, *Writing a Medical Research Manuscript*,
https://doi.org/10.1007/978-3-032-20276-5_29

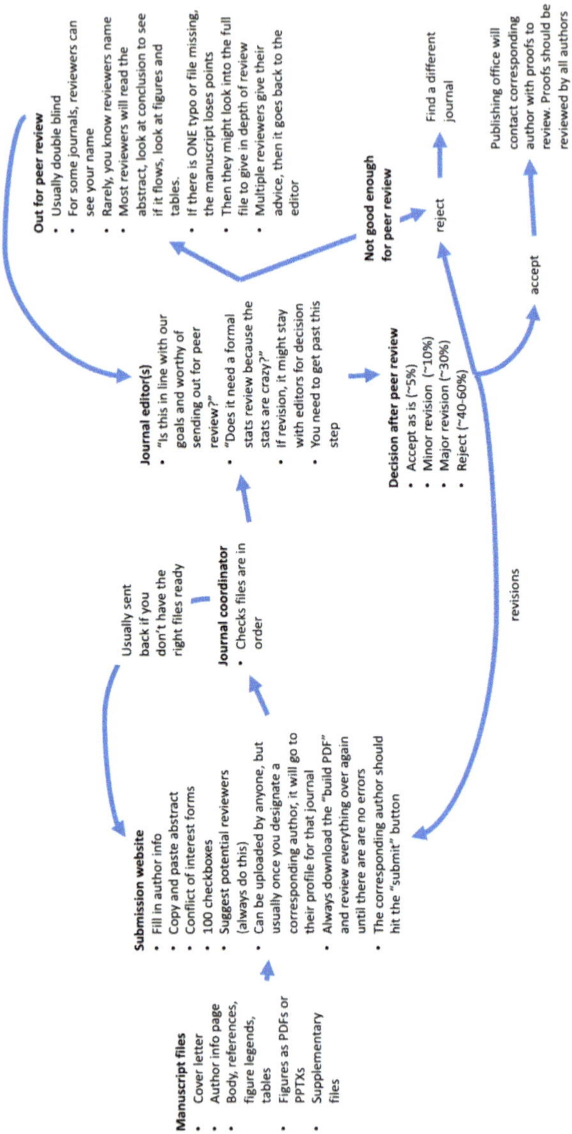

Figure. Submission overview

Keep it submitted algorithm:

- Desk reject → immediate resubmit to a different journal (same day).
- Major revision → revise carefully.
- Methodologic criticism → stop and reassess.

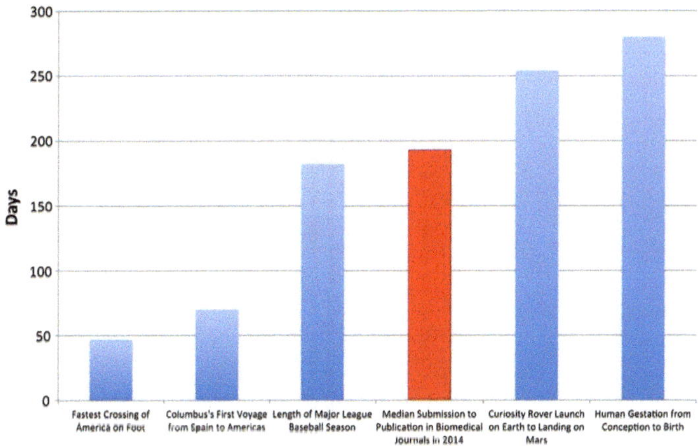

Figure. Publishing a manuscript takes a long time

Most papers will likely get rejected.

- A good benchmark is batting 0.300, i.e., if one-third of papers are going out for review, you are on the right track. Eventually, the paper will be accepted.

How long should you wait before contacting the journal about your paper?

- One to two months is reasonable to send a reminder/check in email. It is unacceptable for journals to hold on to manuscripts for more than three to four months.

Receiving revisions

- Revisions are good. You want revisions and lots of comments from the reviewers. If reviewers hated your paper, they would have left a review of a few sentences and then rejected it.

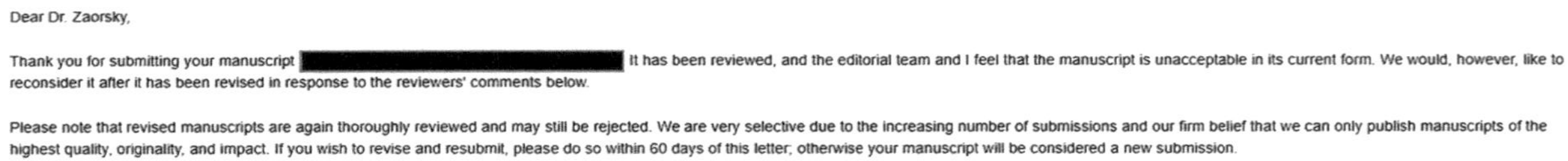

Dear Dr. Zaorsky,

Thank you for submitting your manuscript [redacted] It has been reviewed, and the editorial team and I feel that the manuscript is unacceptable in its current form. We would, however, like to reconsider it after it has been revised in response to the reviewers' comments below.

Please note that revised manuscripts are again thoroughly reviewed and may still be rejected. We are very selective due to the increasing number of submissions and our firm belief that we can only publish manuscripts of the highest quality, originality, and impact. If you wish to revise and resubmit, please do so within 60 days of this letter; otherwise your manuscript will be considered a new submission.

Figure. A favorable email response

30 How Reviewers Read a Paper vs. How Authors Write a Paper

Reviewing vs. Writing a Manuscript

If the editors think your paper is good for review, they will send it to reviewers.

Invited faculty wonder: "Should I accept the invitation to review this research manuscript?"

1. Do you have interest and expertise in this topic?
2. Do you have available time?
3. Would you publish in this journal?

The more you answer "no," the more you should not review it.

If the reviewer chooses to accept, they will next receive the PDF. Reviewers read papers in a different order than authors write the paper. Reviewers focus first on the abstract, tables, and figures, and ask themselves, "would I draw the same conclusion from the data presented?"

N. G. Zaorsky, *Writing a Medical Research Manuscript*,
https://doi.org/10.1007/978-3-032-20276-5_30

How reviewers read a paper:

1. Abstract.
2. Tables and figures.
3. Intro.
4. Methods.
5. +/– Discussion.

How authors write a paper:

1. Hypothesis and prospectus.
2. Tables and figures.
3. Results.
4. Methods.
5. Intro (copy/paste prospectus).
6. Discussion.
7. Abstract.

Most people can tell if a work is good and worth further evaluation after:

- movie: <10 min
- book: <1 chapter
- show: <1 episode
- art, song: <10 s

Similarly, in academics:

- manuscript, grant: <2 min
- abstract: <30 s
- tables, figures: <30 s

If writing a review, provide constructive feedback. Write it as if you are writing to your mentee, to improve their work.

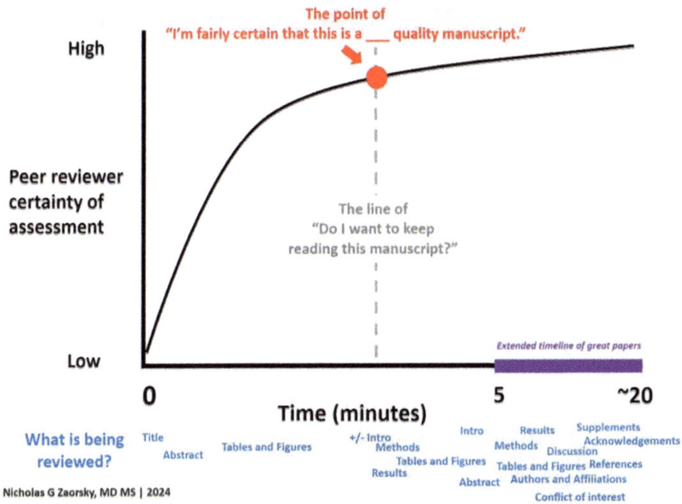

Figure. Time it takes to assess the quality of a medical research manuscript

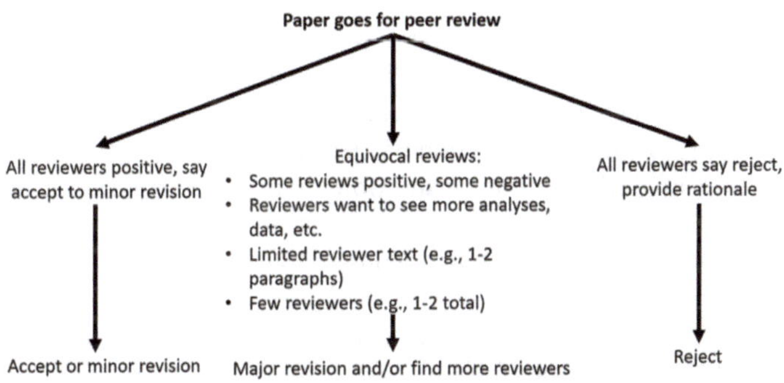

Figure. How editors should deal with various types of reviews. If you are an editor for a journal, receive a submission, and agree with your editorial team to send the paper for peer review, then it is your job to advocate for this paper and give the authors reasonable chances to revise the work (even if reviews are critical)

How to Review a Medical Research Manuscript

- Step 1: Abstract.
  - Intro: states an innovative goal with a clear objective, purpose, aim(s), or hypothesis.
  - Results: uses data (numbers, statistical tests) to address objective, purpose, aim(s), or hypothesis.
    If clinical study, consider PICOS: Patients, Intervention, Control, Outcomes, Study type.
    If basic science, consider cell lines or tissue, drugs, model system, manipulation, controls.
  - Methods: explains how the results were obtained.
    If clinical study, consider: PICOS, CONSORT, PRISMA, REMARK, IRB approval, trial #.
    If basic science, consider: in vitro and in vivo studies.
  - Conclusion: provides summary about the core finding, without overstating findings.
- Step 2: Tables and figures (usually <5 total).
  - High quality.
  - Address the objective, purpose, aim(s), or hypothesis.
  - Interpretable without having to read the text, and ideally without having to read legend.
- Step 3: Results (~2–2.5 double-spaced pages).
  - Sequentially address the objective, purpose, aim(s), or hypothesis.
  - Reference all tables and figures.

Note: If significant issues are present by Step 3, most reviewers will reject the manuscript.

- Step 4: Introduction (~1 double-spaced page).
  - Paragraph 1: What is the overarching problem in medicine?
  - Paragraphs 2–3: What has been done leading up to and necessitating the current study?
  - Final paragraph: Why is the current study done? Objective, purpose, aim(s), or hypothesis?
- Step 5: Methods (~2 double-spaced pages).
  - Are the statistics (study design, endpoint) aligned with the research question?

  - Are the data collection and experimental techniques appropriate and reproducible?
    - Is there an appropriate control?
    - Are confounding variables and bias accounted for?
    - Basic science: 3+ biological replicates performed per experiment?
  - Are statistical models, assumptions, and significance thresholds specified?
- Step 6: Discussion (~1.5–2 double-spaced pages).
  - Paragraph 1:
    - Summarize major problem in medicine, previous attempts to address problem.
    - How this study is novel in its methods/results, putting major finding in perspective.
  - Paragraph 2-n: Discuss findings from objectives, tables, and figures sequentially, in context of existing and future work (similar to an editorial).
  - Final paragraph(s): Limitations, e.g.: selection biases, sample size, missing data, techniques, validity.
- Common errors and red flags, done in conjunction with other sections.
  - No hypothesis, purpose; or work is not novel.
  - Methods cannot be used to address the purpose.
  - Data not quantified, e.g.: no estimates, biostatistics.
  - References not appropriate.
  - Typos, grammar, syntax, abbreviation, significant figure inconsistencies.
  - Ethical concerns, e.g.: financial conflicts of interest, patient care.
  - Conclusions are overstated or are inconsistent throughout manuscript.
  - Appropriate coauthors not involved, e.g.: subspecialists, biostatistician.
  - Needs additional review from a content expert (e.g., biostatistician).
  - Ratio of length of sections above is off (e.g., mostly discussion, limited results).

Writing the Response Letter

31

When to write:

- If you were asked to revise your manuscript by editors.
- Revisions are good. If there are a lot of requested revisions, it usually means the reviewers liked your work. If they didn't like your work, it would be rejected with minimal comments.

Goal of this section:

- To make reasonable changes to your manuscript.
- To show appreciation for reviewers, and agreement between you and the reviewers.
- To avoid conflict between you and reviewers. Conflict leads to rejection.

Background and general advice

- Reviewers usually are not compensated for reviewing; authors should be thankful for reviewers' time.
- Journals typically struggle to find reviewers for any manuscript; the response rate can be <30%.
- Journals request that reviewers evaluate scientific validity and impact on the field.
- Some reviewer comments may be random and pertain to reviewers' own biases.

N. G. Zaorsky, *Writing a Medical Research Manuscript*,
https://doi.org/10.1007/978-3-032-20276-5_31

- The more comments that reviewers leave, the better it is for authors' acceptance potential. Reviewers do not tend to leave lengthy comments for manuscripts they dislike.
- Reviewers typically leave two styles of comments: general overview and gestalt of the manuscript, point-by-point issues they want addressed, or both.
- Even with rejections, reviewers often give guidance to improve the effort for future resubmission.
- If this work was previously submitted, revised, but ultimately rejected, consider providing the point-by-point response letter and your revisions to show that you are actively improving the work.
- General framework for responses: Reviewer comment → Edited comment → Author response → Quoted manuscript change.
- Authors should aim to:
  - First, address the editors stating appreciation for the opportunity to resubmit and that changes were made as recommended by reviewers, and (in select cases) why changes cannot be made.
  - Thank the reviewers for their comments, note if they agree.
  - Provide a point-by-point response for each comment:

    e.g., "REVIEWER COMMENT:"/"AUTHOR RESPONSE:"

    Consider differing colors to make distinction between the comment vs. response.
  - Keep responses respectful and revisions brief.
  - In addition to referencing the manuscript section with changes, copy and paste major changes from text, tables, and figures into the response letter, so the reviewers team does not have to search manuscript manually. After revising, consider: "In the methods/results, we now state:"
  - Ask journal for extension in returning the manuscript for significant revisions, PRN.
- Authors should not:
  - Take reviewer comments personally, argue with reviewers, show conflict, etc.
  - Provide long explanations but change nothing in the manuscript.
  - Provide responses that are long, non-sequitur, respond with what is already stated, etc.

Most reviewer comments and author responses can be categorized into these categories:

Reviewer comment/ request	Comment favorable?	Author action and response
Add statements on ethics, contributions, funding, etc.	Very favorable	Make the edits. Note: this is a comment from the editorial team; it suggests a high likelihood of manuscript acceptance.
Section X is good	Favorable	Thank the reviewer for praising the work.
Make minor edits to grammar, syntax, references, layout, etc.	Favorable	Make the edits.
Table or Figure adds limited information.	Favorable	If authors agree, but the Table/ Figure addresses the purpose, consider moving it to be a supplement. Otherwise, delete.
Discuss something that is already discussed in the manuscript.	Favorable	Add more detail to that section, and/or discuss again in a different section.
Numbers do not match between tables, figures, and text.	Likely favorable	Double check the numbers. Provide inclusion/exclusion criteria. Was a different n used for inclusion vs. analysis?
Make major changes to methods or results.	Depends	Contact the senior author and biostatistics team. If changes cannot be made, explain why. Consider: "This is outside the scope of the current study." "The database contains/does not contain…" "This is the first study to show…; future works will focus on…" "A complementary work focuses on…"
Reject because of perceived issues in methodology, outcome reporting, novelty, etc.	Unfavorable	Unfortunately, this can be a fatal issue for the manuscript and may be due to reviewer bias or poor methods. To avoid these comments, authors should ideally present a hypothesis with appropriate methods.

How to write the letter:

- "Dear {chief editor's name}"
- Common comments and how to address them:

Thank you for your review of our manuscript, "XXX" in your journal. We have reviewed all of the comments below and provided a point-by-point response per your request.

REVIEWER COMMENT: Please integrate XXX in the results.

AUTHOR RESPONSE: Thank you for your helpful comments. We now provide XXX in the results. Specifically, we state:
{copy and paste section from manuscript}

REVIEWER COMMENT: XXX is a garbage variable and should not be reported.

AUTHOR RESPONSE: Thank you for your helpful comments. We agree that XXX is not a good measure of XXX. This variable was reported by the clinical trial / registry / cohort, and there are no other variables available for reporting. We have left the reporting of the variable in case readers are interested in it, and we discuss limitations of this variable in the discussion:
{copy and paste section from manuscript}

REVIEWER COMMENT: XXX is not discussed in the manuscript.

AUTHOR RESPONSE: Thank you for your helpful comments. We now further emphasize discussion of XXX:
{copy and paste section from manuscript}

REVIEWER COMMENT: This needs biostatistics tests, including XXX.

AUTHOR RESPONSE: Thank you for your helpful comments. We have reviewed the work with our biostatistical team (including two PhD level biostatisticians), and {have vs have not} included the tests mentioned because X. We now state in the manuscript:
{copy and paste section from manuscript}

Thank you again for your helpful comments. We believe we have addressed all of the concerns from the editors and reviewers. If you have any other questions, please reach out to us.

Do's and Don'ts of the response letter:

Do:

- Be polite and professional. Consider your reviewers as your colleagues and future collaborators, and treat them as such.
- Respond to all queries and comments. If you don't agree, say so tactfully and explain why.
- Show that you made changes that improved the work. As seen above, copy and paste the changes you made to the manuscript in your response to each question.
- Ask questions if you don't understand a comment. Revisions are like a conversation– you and your reviewers are working together to make final edits to your manuscript. Work with them.

Don't:

- Argue with reviewers.
- Decline to make changes. There are ways around the revision even if you can't make a certain change. In all cases, try to agree with the reviewers, tell them you would ideally do this analysis, but for various reasons, it is not possible. Don't write "we can't do it"; rather, write that "it can't be done." This means that you would love to do it, but various factors preclude you doing it, it's out of everyone's control. For example:
  - "We agree that including this covariate in the analysis would be helpful; unfortunately, not all of the studies included in our work analyzed this variable, so this analysis is not possible. Nonetheless, our work represents the largest analysis on this topic to date around the world, and it builds on all prior analyses."
  - "We are collecting data on this endpoint currently; it will be analyzed and presented in a subsequent manuscript."
  - "The national databases used in this analysis do not include this variable. No national databases around the world contain this variable plus the other variables in our analysis. Thus,

  although it is a limitation, it is relatively small, and our work is still the largest analysis on this topic globally."
  - "The patients declined to provide this variable."
  - "We wanted to collect this variable, and our initial grant application suggested this. However, collection of this variable would have been too costly. The budget for this trial was X, and collecting this variable would have increased it to Y."
- Show conflict.
- Provide non-sequitur responses.

32 Guide to Checking the Prepublication Proof

Background

- The proof is the final prepublished version of your article. It's the last time you get to make changes.
- Some journals have an excellent editorial team that checks all the text, numbers, and references. Other journals are not as meticulous and could make changes that negatively affect the quality of your work, e.g., uploading low-quality figures, even though you had provided high-quality rasters and vectors.
- You should email the proof to all coauthors ASAP and ask for edits.
  - "Hello team, here is our proof. Please review and send comments to me/the first author/the senior author within the next week."
  - If you need more time for you and authors to review, respond to the publisher with an estimated date when you will have it back.
- Consider asking to check a revised version of the proof if significant edits needed (e.g., figures are low quality).

Checklist

- Address author queries from editorial team.
- Read through the entire paper once.
- Author names, spelling.

N. G. Zaorsky, *Writing a Medical Research Manuscript*,
https://doi.org/10.1007/978-3-032-20276-5_32

- Author affiliations.
- ORCIDs for authors (if being used).
- Number of authors (make sure you are not missing anyone).
- Funding, support, and potential conflicts of interest.
- Tables and figures:
  - High quality (no blurry images).
  - Number of each table and figure matches where it is cited in the manuscript.
  - Number of tables and figures listed in the manuscript = number of tables and figures uploaded.
  - Values add up correctly, e.g.:
    - PRISMA, CONSORT diagrams.
    - Table sums.
- Aesthetics: ideally, the abstract, figures + legends, tables, should not spill a few lines on subsequent pages.
- Obtain approval of the proof from all coauthors.
  - Check that references are correctly numbered and linked.
  - Check corresponding author information.

How to Update Publications and Abstracts in Your CV

33

N. G. Zaorsky, *Writing a Medical Research Manuscript*,
https://doi.org/10.1007/978-3-032-20276-5_33

Step 1: Organize your CV into the sections below

Step 2: During regular intervals (e.g., as you travel to/from a meeting, yearly evaluation), update the CV:

Section in your CV	Where to find	How to get to your CV	Example
Publications	PubMed	Search your name, sort by most recent, select, copy, paste.	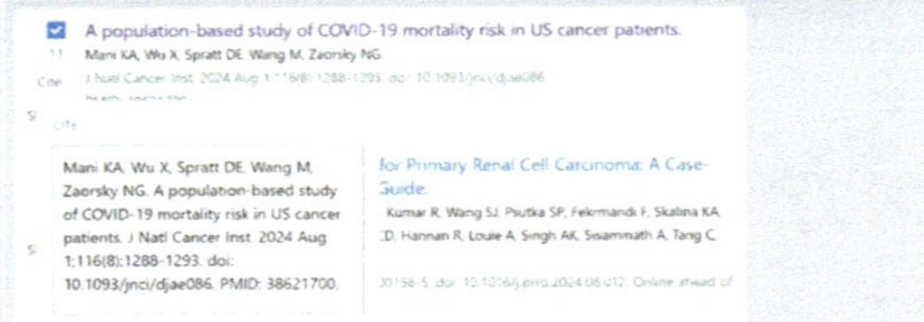
└ Original research			
└ Review articles			
└ Invited commentary			
└ Case reports			
└ Other			
Abstracts, presentations			
└ National, international	Google scholar	Set up profile. Profile is updated automatically. Sort by most recent. Check off recent abstracts, export to CSV, copy, paste. Modify formatting as needed.	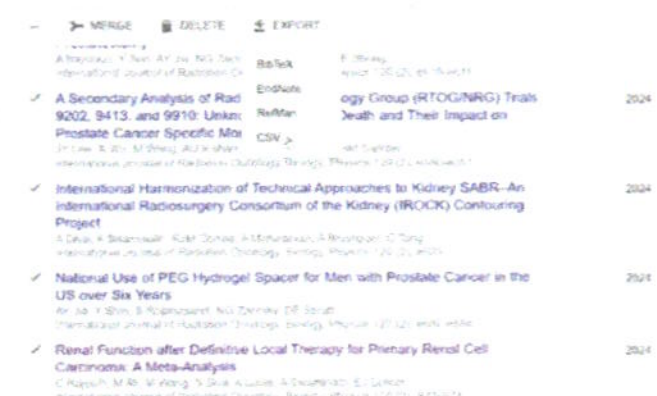
└ Regional, departmental	N/A	Type manually immediately after you deliver it.	

Figure. How to update publications and abstracts in your CV

34 Publicizing Your Work

Social Media (Twitter, LinkedIn, etc.)

- In an age of algorithms, perhaps the easiest way to reach a wide audience of readers is through social media.
- Share a link to your paper, along with a short synopsis of the aims and main findings.
- Share key figures from your publication.
- Engage with other users. Ask/answer questions, use hashtags, and build a network to help your research reach a wider audience.
- General advice for your tweets:
  - Quantify your findings.
  - Use open-ended questions.
  - Avoid medical jargon.
- Tag coauthors, institutions, and journals when appropriate.
- Include the DOI or direct article link in every post.
- Share conference presentations or visual abstracts to broaden reach.

Institution

- Most institutions have a public relations team that shares news and accomplishments of its faculty both internally and externally.
- Ask if they will share your research on internal newsletters, or if they will highlight your work on institutional social media accounts.

N. G. Zaorsky, *Writing a Medical Research Manuscript*, https://doi.org/10.1007/978-3-032-20276-5_34

35 How to Write a Research Abstract for Presentation at a Meeting

Title:

- Short statement that integrates the purpose, findings, and/or conclusion
- ***Common errors:***
  - ***Esoteric abbreviations.***
  - ***Focuses on methods.***
  - ***States interpretation of the results.***

Introduction/background:

- Brief, pertinent background, highlighting the missing knowledge gap. Note: for most abstracts, reviewers will already have basic understanding of the field.
- Purpose, hypothesis, aim, or objective of the current study.
- ***Common errors:***
  - ***Too much background.***
  - ***No hypothesis or purpose; or hypothesis is not novel.***

Methods:

- What was done to address the purpose? How was this done?
  - Are the statistics (study design, endpoint, etc.) aligned with the research question?
  - Bias: how are confounding bias, selection bias, etc. accounted for?

N. G. Zaorsky, *Writing a Medical Research Manuscript*,
https://doi.org/10.1007/978-3-032-20276-5_35

- If clinical, consider:
  - Population: What were the inclusion and exclusion criteria? How many patients? Time frame?
  - Intervention: What was the treatment? Pertinent details?
  - Control: Was there a control or reference group?
  - Outcomes: What was the primary endpoint? In general, the most important measures for patients: *quantity* of life (overall survival) and *quality* of life (e.g., patient reported outcomes, toxicity). Most other measures are surrogates. If using a surrogate, how is it defined?
  - Setting: Prospective, retrospective, randomized, case control?
- If basic science, consider:
  - Setting: in vitro, in vivo, in silico, etc.
  - Interventions/experiments: cell lines or tissue/mice used; drugs or treatments; controls.
  - # of times each experiment was repeated and the sample size (*n*).
- ***Common errors:***
  - ***Methods cannot be used to assess the purpose.***
  - ***Insufficient biostatistics.***
  - ***Unnecessary details; elaborates on everything done, taking up characters.***
  - ***Provides spillover from the background or results.***

Results:

- General
  - The most important and usually the longest part of the abstract.
  - Use numbers and statistical tests to present the data.
  - Consistency in significant figures (rarely needs >2–3 sig figs, going to 0.1%, etc.).
  - Quantitative: list specific estimates, confidence intervals, *p*-values, ratios, risks, *n* (%).
  - Depending on the study type and data, consider:

    For non-normally distributed data (most medical data), list medians and IQRs.

    For normally distributed data (most basic science data), list means and SDs or SEMs.

  - If presenting comparative point estimates, list the 95% CI and/or *p*-value. If low on characters, cut the *p*-values, but not the CIs.
  - Use correct estimates in reporting and interpretation:
    Relative: HRs, ORs, RRs.
    Absolute: what is the overall difference? Are differences *clinically* meaningful?
  - Consider using a table to list results (if conference abstract submission allows).
- Sentences 1–2
  - Provide descriptive statistics.
  - If clinical, consider pertinent results as they relate to methods: eligibility, inclusion, exclusion; time of study; location of study; patient characteristics; treatment.
  - If basic science: controls used, baseline expression of protein or phenomena of interest in cell lines, animal model, or tissue analyzed.
- Sentences 3–5
  - Basic science: list experiments in logical order.
  - Translational: In vitro, in vivo, in patients.
  - Clinical: outcomes, toxicities, prognostication, prediction.
  - Consider study limitations.
- ***Common errors:***
  - ***Shorter than other sections.***
  - ***Insufficient quantification of the data: no estimates, CIs, p-values, no absolute or relative info.***
  - ***Out of logical order.***
  - ***Repeats info from methods.***

Conclusion:
- Addresses purpose, aim, goal, or hypothesis, relating to results.
- Provides a single core take–home message.
- Sometimes mentions potential implications, without overstating findings.
- ***Common errors:***
  - ***Does not address the hypothesis or purpose.***
  - ***Presents known background, information that should be in the intro.***

- *Overstates findings, discusses possible things that could happen with the data.*
- *Longer than one to two sentences.*

Common errors throughout entire abstract:

- *Grammar, spelling, syntax: Jumping tense. Typos. Abbreviation inundation: acronyms should be used sparingly (one to three terms), be consistent, be routinely used in the literature (e.g., HIV, AIDS), decrease word count.*
- *Significant figure issues.*
- *"Missing the forest for the trees": presenting all subgroup estimates, all time points, p-values, CIs, etc., rather than focusing on pertinent estimates.*
- *Fishing expedition: performing an analysis that looks for any associations. No correction for multiple comparisons (e.g., Bonferroni).*
- *Starting sentences with the word "this"/Subject is unclear.*
- *"Longer/better" outcome, without absolute and relative quantification.*
- *"Some…": "…of the [patients/sample]"; "…improvement in outcomes."*
- *Length of sections is not: results > methods > conclusion or intro/purpose.*

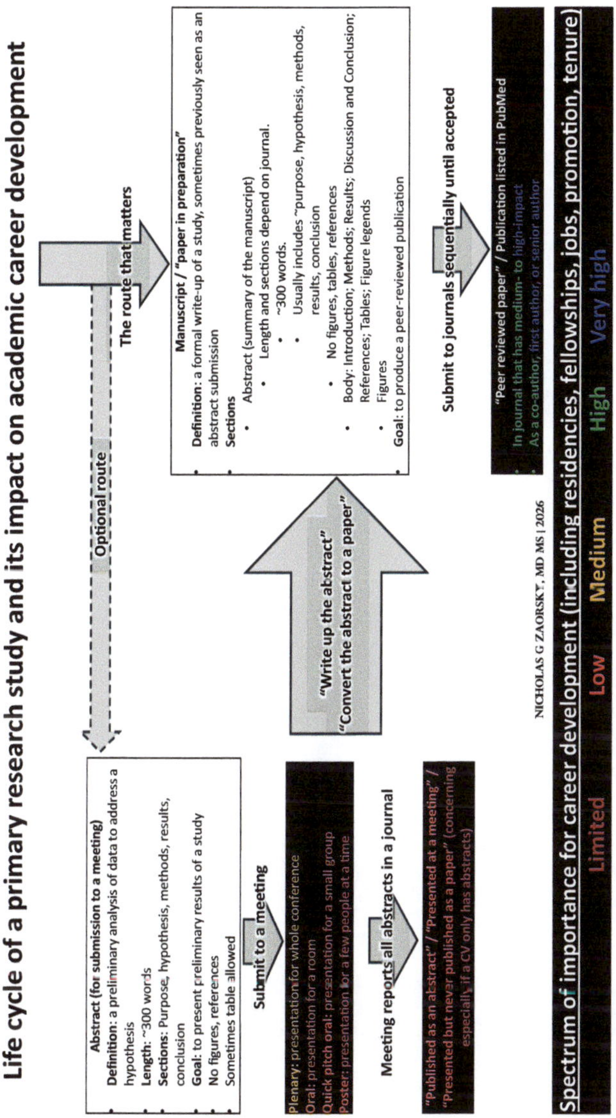
Life cycle of a primary research study and its impact on academic career development
Abstract (for submission to a meeting)
Definition: a preliminary analysis of data to address a hypothesis
Length: ~300 words
Sections: Purpose, hypothesis, methods, results, conclusion
Goal: to present preliminary results of a study
No figures, references
Sometimes table allowed
Optional route
The route that matters
Manuscript / "paper in preparation"
Definition: a formal write-up of a study, sometimes previously seen as an abstract submission
Sections
Abstract (summary of the manuscript)
Length and sections depend on journal.
~300 words.
Usually includes ~purpose, hypothesis, methods, results, conclusion
No figures, tables, references
Body: Introduction; Methods; Results; Discussion and Conclusion; References; Tables; Figure legends
Figures
Goal: to produce a peer-reviewed publication
Submit to a meeting
Plenary: presentation for whole conference
Oral: presentation for a room
Quick pitch oral: presentation for a small group
Poster: presentation for a few people at a time
"Write up the abstract"
"Convert the abstract to a paper"
Submit to journals sequentially until accepted
Meeting reports all abstracts in a journal
"Published as an abstract" / "Presented at a meeting" /
"Presented but never published as a paper" (concerning especially if a CV only has abstracts)
"Peer reviewed paper" / Publication listed in PubMed
In journal that has medium- to high-impact
As a co-author, first author, or senior author
NICHOLAS G ZAORSKY, MD MS | 2026
Spectrum of importance for career development (including residencies, fellowships, jobs, promotion, tenure)
Limited
Low
Medium
High
Very high

36 How to Give an Oral Presentation at a Meeting

- Send your presentation to many people for comments/feedback. Always send to coauthors, senior author, discussant (if there is one).
  - Also consider other specialists in your field, colleagues, family/friends, who can give you more blunt advice as outsiders.
- Practice your talk many times over until it flows smoothly.
  - As a resident, you may need to practice it more than ten times.
  - Your goal is to have no filler words (e.g., "ummmm"). Have people count your umms and report after you finish.
- Your name and title will be presented before you go on stage, so you don't need to present these.
- General slide etiquette.
  - The header usually summarizes a core message.
  - Aim for seven words per line, seven lines per slide.
  - Try to avoid text-only slides.
  - Do not read verbatim.
- Most oral presentations are about 10 min long, with 8 min of presentation and 2 min of Q/A.
  - In the 8 min, aim for:

    1 min title, thanks, disclosure.
    1 min background/objectives.
    1 min methods.
    4 min results.
    1 min conclusion.

N. G. Zaorsky, *Writing a Medical Research Manuscript*,
https://doi.org/10.1007/978-3-032-20276-5_36

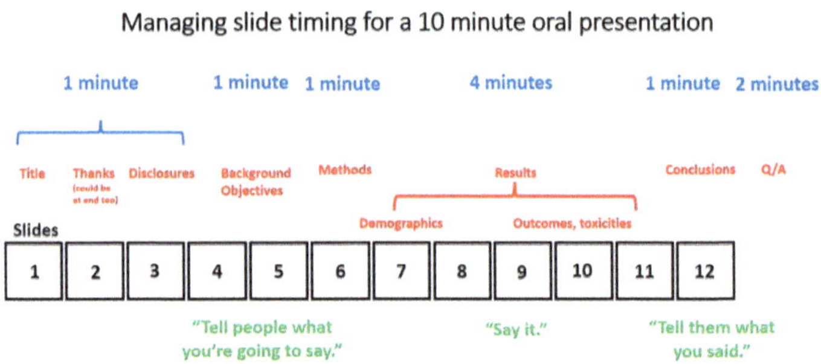

Figure. Overview of a 7–10 min oral presentation of your project

- Avoid background photos and excessive logos, badges, etc. because they can make it difficult to interpret the contents of the slide.
- If presenting a table or figure, slow down and explain what it shows:
  - "The rows/columns show…"
  - "The x-axis is… /the y-axis is…"
  - "This is a Kaplan–Meier plot of…"
  - "The colors represent…"
  - "The size of each point correlates with…"
  - "We are coplotting…"
- If you are at a subspecialty meeting, you usually do not have to explain common abbreviations.
- If you copy and paste a figure, double check the formatting so it is high quality.
  - No grainy images.
  - Consider copy/pasting over the axes to better display the text.
  - No red squiggly underlines.
- If you have a table, please make it a table in your slideshow. Don't copy and paste an image of a table, especially with typos. It will look sloppy.
- If you provide a reference, consider just listing the first author/organization, journal, year. You could provide a screenshot of the title as needed, but it's rarely necessary to provide a screenshot of title + authors + journal. Otherwise, the image will take up too much space.

- Your figures are often the most important part of the presentation.
- As you advance in your career, it will take less time to revise a presentation and improve its quality. Most people (including residents and many faculty) need to deliver the presentation multiple times before the conference.
- How to handle questions from the audience:
  - Repeat the question for the audience before answering.
  - If unsure of the answer, acknowledge the limitation honestly.
  - Keep answers brief; offer to discuss further offline if needed.

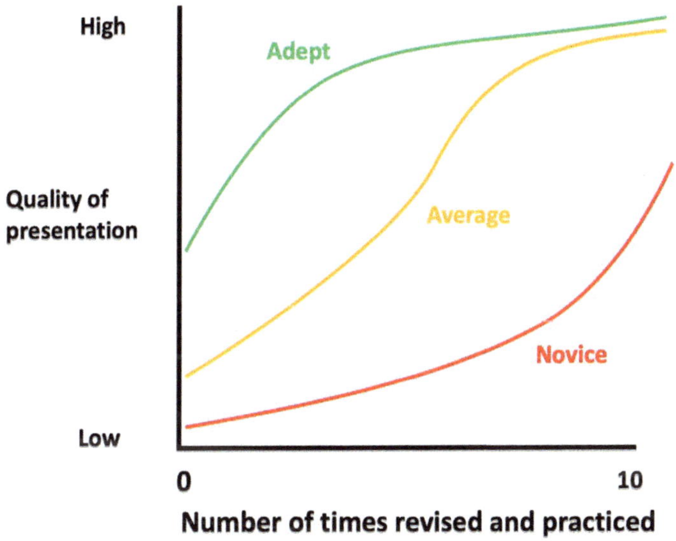

Figure. Quality of your presentation vs number of times revised and practiced

- Have a core message you repeat for the audience.
  - Tell people what you're going to say.
  - Say it.
  - Tell them what you said.
- The abstract and the oral presentation should have relatively similar content.
  - You don't want to be presenting data contrasting what you initially submitted.

37 How to Pack for a Professional/Medical Research Conference

N. G. Zaorsky, *Writing a Medical Research Manuscript*,
https://doi.org/10.1007/978-3-032-20276-5_37

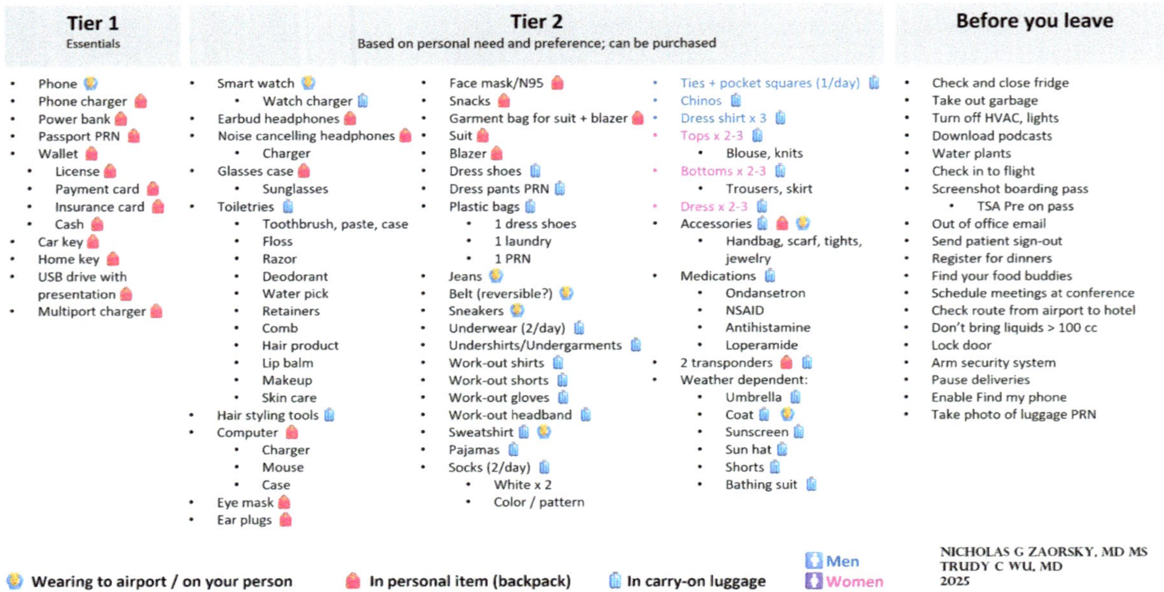

Figure. How to pack for a professional conference

Suggested Readings

1. Aga SS, Nissar S. Essential guide to manuscript writing for academic dummies: an editor's perspective. Biochem Res Int. 2022;2022:1492058. https://doi.org/10.1155/2022/1492058. PMID: 36092536; PMCID: PMC9458406.
2. Kotz D, Cals JW. Effective writing and publishing scientific papers—part I: how to get started. J Clin Epidemiol. 2013;66(4):397. https://doi.org/10.1016/j.jclinepi.2013.01.002. PMID: 23452726.
3. Cals JW, Kotz D. Effective writing and publishing scientific papers, part II: title and abstract. J Clin Epidemiol. 2013;66(6):585. https://doi.org/10.1016/j.jclinepi.2013.01.005. Epub 2013 Feb 19. PMID: 23434329.
4. Cals JW, Kotz D. Effective writing and publishing scientific papers, part III: introduction. J Clin Epidemiol. 2013;66(7):702. https://doi.org/10.1016/j.jclinepi.2013.01.004. Epub 2013 Mar 13. PMID: 23497856.
5. Kotz D, Cals JW. Effective writing and publishing scientific papers, part IV: methods. J Clin Epidemiol. 2013;66(8):817. https://doi.org/10.1016/j.jclinepi.2013.01.003. Epub 2013 Feb 19. PMID: 23434330.
6. Kotz D, Cals JW. Effective writing and publishing scientific papers, part V: results. J Clin Epidemiol. 2013;66(9):945. https://doi.org/10.1016/j.jclinepi.2013.04.003. Epub 2013 Jun 19. PMID: 23791158.
7. Cals JW, Kotz D. Effective writing and publishing scientific papers, part VI: discussion. J Clin Epidemiol. 2013;66(10):1064. https://doi.org/10.1016/j.jclinepi.2013.04.017. PMID: 23993311.
8. Kotz D, Cals JW. Effective writing and publishing scientific papers, part VII: tables and figures. J Clin Epidemiol. 2013;66(11):1197. https://doi.org/10.1016/j.jclinepi.2013.04.016. Epub 2013 Aug 17. PMID: 23958377.
9. Cals JW, Kotz D. Effective writing and publishing scientific papers, part VIII: references. J Clin Epidemiol. 2013;66(11):1198. https://doi.org/10.1016/j.jclinepi.2013.06.015. PMID: 24079642.
10. Cals JW, Kotz D. Effective writing and publishing scientific papers, part IX: authorship. J Clin Epidemiol. 2013;66(12):1319. https://doi.org/10.1016/j.jclinepi.2013.08.006. Epub 2013 Oct 26. PMID: 24369122.

N. G. Zaorsky, *Writing a Medical Research Manuscript*,
https://doi.org/10.1007/978-3-032-20276-5

11. Cals JW, Kotz D. Effective writing and publishing scientific papers, part X: choice of journal. J Clin Epidemiol. 2014;67(1):3. https://doi.org/10.1016/j.jclinepi.2013.09.014. Epub 2013 Oct 31. PMID: 24183607.
12. Kotz D, Cals JW. Effective writing and publishing scientific papers, part XI: submitting a paper. J Clin Epidemiol. 2014;67(2):123. https://doi.org/10.1016/j.jclinepi.2013.10.004. Erratum in: J Clin Epidemiol. 2015 Sep;68(9):1115. PMID: 24377385.
13. Kotz D, Cals JW. Effective writing and publishing scientific papers, part XII: responding to reviewers. J Clin Epidemiol. 2014;67(3):243. https://doi.org/10.1016/j.jclinepi.2013.10.003. Epub 2014 Jan 9. PMID: 24411072.
14. Chopra V, Edelson DP, Saint S. A piece of my mind. Mentorship malpractice. JAMA. 2016;315(14):1453–4. https://doi.org/10.1001/jama.2015.18884. PMID: 27115263.
15. Cushman M. How I respond to peer reviewer comments. Res Pract Thromb Haemost. 2023;7(2):100120. https://doi.org/10.1016/j.rpth.2023.100120. PMID: 37063759; PMCID: PMC10099302.
16. DeCastro R, Sambuco D, Ubel PA, Stewart A, Jagsi R. Batting 300 is good: perspectives of faculty researchers and their mentors on rejection, resilience, and persistence in academic medical careers. Acad Med. 2013;88(4):497–504. https://doi.org/10.1097/ACM.0b013e318285f3c0. PMID: 23425991; PMCID: PMC3645975.
17. Deng B. Papers with shorter titles get more citations. Nature [Internet]. 2015 [cited 2025 Aug 22]. https://doi.org/10.1038/nature.2015.18246.
18. Forero DA, Lopez-Leon S, Perry G. A brief guide to the science and art of writing manuscripts in biomedicine. J Transl Med. 2020;18(1):425. https://doi.org/10.1186/s12967-020-02596-2. PMID: 33167977; PMCID: PMC7653709.
19. Hammond DA, Rech MA. A "how-to" guide for effectively writing a publishable research manuscript. J Am Coll Clin Pharm. 2020;3:818–24. https://doi.org/10.1002/jac5.1190.
20. Huecker MR, Shreffler J. How to write and publish a scientific manuscript. Treasure Island (FL): StatPearls Publishing; 2025. 2022 Oct 31. StatPearls [Internet]. PMID: 33232064.
21. Golden SH, Bass EB. Validity of meta-analysis in diabetes: meta-analysis is an indispensable tool in evidence synthesis. Diabetes Care. 2013;36(10):3368–73. https://doi.org/10.2337/dc13-1196. PMID: 24065845; PMCID: PMC3781512.
22. Grant MJ, Booth A. A typology of reviews: an analysis of 14 review types and associated methodologies. Health Info Libr J. 2009;26(2):91–108. https://doi.org/10.1111/j.1471-1842.2009.00848.x. PMID: 19490148.
23. Hanna M. How to write better medical papers. Cham, Switzerland: Springer; 2019.
24. Hardman TC, Krentz AJ, Wierzbicki AS. Ten tips for promoting your research. Cardiovascular Endocrinology & Metabolism. 2020;9(1):30–35. https://doi.org/10.1097/XCE.0000000000000191.

25. Kliewer MA. Writing it up: a step-by-step guide to publication for beginning investigators. AJR Am J Roentgenol. 2005;185(3):591–6. https://doi.org/10.2214/ajr.185.3.01850591. PMID: 16120904.
26. Lawrence TS. Writing a research paper. Int J Radiat Oncol Biol Phys. 2020;106(4):674–6. https://doi.org/10.1016/j.ijrobp.2019.12.005. PMID: 32092340.
27. Liumbruno GM, Velati C, Pasqualetti P, Franchini M. How to write a scientific manuscript for publication. Blood Transfus. 2013;11(2):217–26. https://doi.org/10.2450/2012.0247-12. Epub 2012 Dec 21. PMID: 23356975; PMCID: PMC3626472.
28. Lehrer EJ, Wang M, Sun Y, Zaorsky NG. An introduction to meta-analysis. Int J Radiat Oncol Biol Phys. 2023;115(3):564–71. https://doi.org/10.1016/j.ijrobp.2022.07.1831. PMID: 36725168.
29. Lubker R. Guides: literature reviews (health sciences): what is a literature review? [Internet]. [cited 2025 July 21]. Available from: https://musc.libguides.com/reviews/intro.
30. Mensh B, Kording K. Ten simple rules for structuring papers. PLoS Comput Biol. 2017;13(9):e1005619. https://doi.org/10.1371/journal.pcbi.1005619. Erratum in: PLoS Comput Biol. 2017 Nov 9;13(11):e1005830. 10.1371/journal.pcbi.1005830. PMID: 28957311; PMCID: PMC5619685.
31. Page MJ, McKenzie JE, Bossuyt PM, Boutron I, Hoffmann TC, Mulrow CD, Shamseer L, Tetzlaff JM, Akl EA, Brennan SE, Chou R, Glanville J, Grimshaw JM, Hróbjartsson A, Lalu MM, Li T, Loder EW, Mayo-Wilson E, McDonald S, McGuinness LA, Stewart LA, Thomas J, Tricco AC, Welch VA, Whiting P, Moher D. The PRISMA 2020 statement: an updated guideline for reporting systematic reviews. BMJ. 2021;372:n71. https://doi.org/10.1136/bmj.n71. PMID: 33782057; PMCID: PMC8005924.
32. Palma DA, Olson R, Harrow S, Gaede S, Louie AV, Haasbeek C, Mulroy L, Lock M, Rodrigues GB, Yaremko BP, Schellenberg D, Ahmad B, Griffioen G, Senthi S, Swaminath A, Kopek N, Liu M, Moore K, Currie S, Bauman GS, Warner A, Senan S. Stereotactic ablative radiotherapy versus standard of care palliative treatment in patients with oligometastatic cancers (SABR-COMET): a randomised, phase 2, open-label trial. Lancet. 2019;393(10185):2051–8. https://doi.org/10.1016/S0140-6736(18)32487-5. Epub 2019 Apr 11. PMID: 30982687.
33. Recommendations for a Classification of AI use in academic manuscript preparation. STM Association; 2025 Sept 22. Available from: https://stm-assoc.org/document/recommendations-for-a-classification-of-ai-use-in-academic-manuscript-preparation/.
34. Sambunjak D, Straus SE, Marusić A. Mentoring in academic medicine: a systematic review. JAMA. 2006;296(9):1103–15. https://doi.org/10.1001/jama.296.9.1103. PMID: 16954490.
35. Sambunjak D, Straus SE, Marusic A. A systematic review of qualitative research on the meaning and characteristics of mentoring in academic medicine. J Gen Intern Med. 2010;25(1):72–8. https://doi.org/10.1007/

s11606-009-1165-8. Epub 2009 Nov 19. PMID: 19924490; PMCID: PMC2811592.
36. Setiati S, Harimurti K. Writing for scientific medical manuscript: a guide for preparing manuscript submitted to biomedical journals. Acta Med Indones. 2007;39(1):50–5. PMID: 17297211.
37. Stiell IG, Canadian EM Writing Group. Guide to writing and publishing a scientific manuscript: part 1-the structure. CJEM. 2022;24(2):117–9. https://doi.org/10.1007/s43678-021-00241-5. Epub 2021 Dec 21. PMID: 34932211; PMCID: PMC8904337.
38. Stiell IG, Canadian E. M. Writing Group. Guide to writing and publishing a scientific manuscript: part 2-the process. CJEM. 2022;24(2):120–2. https://doi.org/10.1007/s43678-021-00242-4. Epub 2022 Jan 10. PMID: 35006583.
39. Straus SE, Johnson MO, Marquez C, Feldman MD. Characteristics of successful and failed mentoring relationships: a qualitative study across two academic health centers. Acad Med. 2013;88(1):82–9. https://doi.org/10.1097/ACM.0b013e31827647a0. PMID: 23165266; PMCID: PMC3665769.
40. Straus SE, Straus C, Tzanetos K. International campaign to revitalise academic medicine. Career choice in academic medicine: systematic review. J Gen Intern Med. 2006;21(12):1222–9. https://doi.org/10.1111/j.1525-1497.2006.00599.x. PMID: 17105520; PMCID: PMC1924755.
41. Stroup DF, Berlin JA, Morton SC, Olkin I, Williamson GD, Rennie D, Moher D, Becker BJ, Sipe TA, Thacker SB. Meta-analysis of observational studies in epidemiology: a proposal for reporting. Meta-analysis of observational studies in epidemiology (MOOSE) group. JAMA. 2000;283(15):2008–12. https://doi.org/10.1001/jama.283.15.2008. PMID: 10789670.
42. Vickers AJ, Assel M, Dunn RL, MacLennan G, Walz J, Gratzke C, Rouprêt M, Briganti A. How to write a response to reviewers. Eur Urol. 2025;87(5):497–500. https://doi.org/10.1016/j.eururo.2024.12.014. Epub 2025 Jan 6. PMID: 39765388.
43. Yoo JH. Defining the Boundaries of AI Use in Scientific Writing: A Comparative Review of Editorial Policies. J Korean Med Sci. 2025 Jun 16;40(23):e187. doi: 10.3346/jkms.2025.40.e187. PMID: 40524628; PMCID: PMC12170296.
44. Yukawa M, Gansky SA, O'Sullivan P, Teherani A, Feldman MD. A new mentor evaluation tool: evidence of validity. PLoS One. 2020;15(6):e0234345 https://doi.org/10.1371/journal.pone.0234345. PMID: 32544185; PMCID: PMC7297334.
45. Zaorsky NG, O'Brien E, Mardini J, Lehrer EJ, Holliday E, Weisman CS. Publication productivity and academic rank in medicine: a systematic review and meta-analysis. Acad Med. 2020;95(8):1274–82. https://doi.org/10.1097/ACM.0000000000003185. PMID: 32028299.
46. Zerzan JT, Hess R, Schur E, Phillips RS, Rigotti N. Making the most of mentors: a guide for mentees. Acad Med. 2009;84(1):140–4. https://doi.org/10.1097/ACM.0b013e3181906e8f. PMID: 19116494.

Index

N. G. Zaorsky, *Writing a Medical Research Manuscript*, https://doi.org/10.1007/978-3-032-20276-5

MIX
Papier aus verantwortungsvollen Quellen
Paper from responsible sources
FSC® C105338

If you have any concerns about our products,
you can contact us on
ProductSafety@springernature.com

In case Publisher is established outside the EU,
the EU authorized representative is:
Springer Nature Customer Service Center GmbH
Europaplatz 3, 69115 Heidelberg, Germany

Printed by Libri Plureos GmbH
in Hamburg, Germany